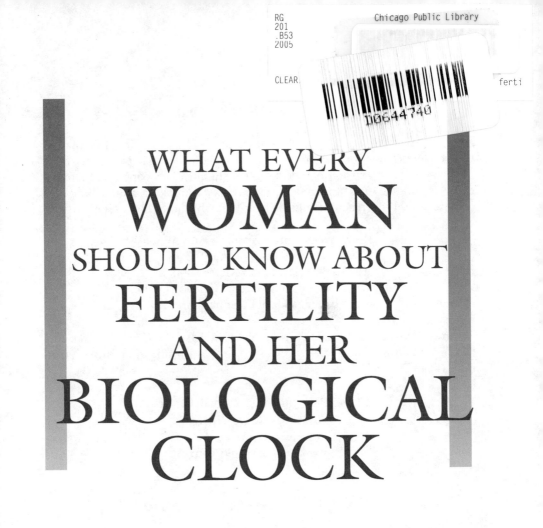

WHAT EVERY
WOMAN
SHOULD KNOW ABOUT
FERTILITY
AND HER
BIOLOGICAL
CLOCK

By

CARA BIRRITTIERI

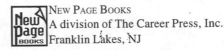
NEW PAGE BOOKS
A division of The Career Press, Inc.
Franklin Lakes, NJ

WHAT EVERY WOMAN SHOULD KNOW ABOUT
FERTILITY AND HER BIOLOGICAL CLOCK
EDITED AND TYPESET BY KRISTEN PARKES
Cover design by Lu Rossman/Digi Dog Design
Printed in the U.S.A. by Book-mart Press

To order this title, please call toll-free 1-800-CAREER-1 (NJ and Canada: 201-848-0310) to order using VISA or MasterCard, or for further information on books from Career Press.

The Career Press, Inc., 3 Tice Road, PO Box 687,
Franklin Lakes, NJ 07417
www.careerpress.com
www.newpagebooks.com

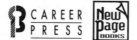

Library of Congress Cataloging-in-Publication Data

Birrittieri, Cara, 1959-
   What every woman should know about fertility and her biological clock /
Cara Birrittieri.
      p. cm.
   Includes bibliographical references and index.
   ISBN 1-56414-735-5 (pbk.)
      1. Infertility, Female. 2. Reproductive health. 3. Fertility, Human. 4. Human reproductive technology. I. Title.

RG201.B53 2005
618.1'78--dc22

                                                          2004055951

Dedicated to
A.J. and Victoria Maria—
my miracle children.

ACKNOWLEDGMENTS

This book could never have been written had it not been for all the support and encouragement from the reproductive medicine community. Individual physicians, researchers, as well as professional and advocacy groups all provided their time, contacts, and expertise. The public affairs department of the American Society for Reproductive Medicine was most helpful with contacting its members and other experts, and providing access to the journal *Fertility and Sterility*. Much thanks to Sean Tipton, Eleanor Nicoll, and Amelia Lambert for all their support and timely assistance. Though this is not meant to be an infertility book, the advocacy group RESOLVE: The National Infertility Association, and its Massachusetts chapter, RESOLVE of the Baystate, provided a tremendous amount of information, and dozens of its members related their personal stories.

Many thanks to the most important doctor I have ever had—my reproductive endocrinologist. Not only did he help me every step of the way with my own cranky clock, and finally guide me toward conceiving my precious daughter, but his willingness and ability to answer my many pointed and sometimes provocative questions, inspired me to press on with this project. Other individuals who were critical to compiling the information and messages here include David Keefe, M.D., who provided his expertise, and generous interviewing time; as well as Jonathan Tilly, Ph.D.; Patricia McShane, M.D.; Zev Rosenwaks, M.D.; Michael Soules, M.D.; Howard Jones Jr., M.D.; James Grifo, M.D.; Alan DeCherney, M.D.; Richard Paulson, M.D.; Gianpiero Palermo, M.D.; Kutluk Oktay, M.D.; Thomas Toth, M.D.; Robert Stillman, M.D.; Michael Feinman, M.D.; Bradford Kolb, M.D.; Michael Fakih, M.D.; Jeffery Boldt, M.D.; Marcelle Cedars, M.D.; Louis O'Dea, M.D.; Barry Behr, Ph.D.; Mark Hughes, M.D.; Ph.D., Roger Gosden, Ph.D., Ds.C.; Machelle Seibel, M.D.; Hope Ricciotti, M.D.; Laura Riley, M.D.; Joseph Sanfilippo, M.D.; Diane Clapp, B.S.N., R.N.; Alice Domar, Ph.D.; Linda Applegarth, Ed.D.; Craig Packer, Ph.D.; Victoria Girard, J.D.; Paul Wolpe, Ph.D.; George Annas, J.D., M.P.H.; and Michael Grodin, M.D.

In addition, several people provided personal as well as professional inspiration, special thanks to Kristen Auclair, Lee Rubin Collins, Christy Jones, Lindsay Nohr, Connie Jarowey, Gina Cella, Andrea Grealish, Carol Lesser, Kim Summers, Gail Marrella, Colleen Cavanaugh, Barbara Fischer, Meghan Slattery, Sharon Saarinen, Ellen Glazer, Peg Beck, Kristen Parkes, Randy Olson, and David Ahrendts.

Of course, a project like this would never be possible without the support of friends and family. So thanks to all those who took the time to help with my son while my husband was away, as well as my mother for all her babysitting duties, my sisters, brother, and in-laws for their constant support. And thanks is an understatement when it comes to my husband, Jackson, who never doubted the importance of this project, championed its cause, and encouraged my efforts, especially when I needed it most.

CONTENTS

INTRODUCTION

As soon as I heard that first cry, I cried. The weight of the world finally lifted off my shoulders when my little girl breathed her first breath. All the turmoil, trauma, and devastating disappointments of my infertility flashed through my mind, and washed instantly away when I knew I would at last become a mother again. At that moment, all that mattered was this tiny new life. A life that was first expected, then dreamed about, then tormented over, and then fought for in ways I can never truly express to anyone. In fact, so much of my journey to having my second child is beyond words that I rarely even bother to talk about it. What I share with you now and with anyone that is interested enough to listen are important facts mostly about what did not happen and why, as well as what I learned that helped me to finally arrive at this incredible pivotal moment in my life.

Somewhere between dreaming about my baby and tormenting over my inability to conceive her, I immersed myself in the study of a certain aspect of reproductive medicine. The experts have all kinds of names for it—diminished ovarian reserve, advanced maternal age, age-related infertility, pre-perimenopause—they sound very antiseptic, don't they? We all are very well aware of what causes this condition every woman goes through whether they realize it or not, though we don't have any fancy name for it. It's simply the *biological clock*. It's a term that strikes fear into the heart of most women, especially those without children who have already passed the age of 30. Like most clocks, this one runs on it's own power source, and we can't ever be certain that the time we see, or should I say *assume*, is correct. Once the power source fades, the clock may still run, but it can fool us into believing we have more time to get where we want to go, when the deadline may have quietly passed us by. I came to understand all there is to know about these tricky biological clocks just a little bit too late.

However, as my appetite for information expanded, I realized I was gathering information that nobody else had previously compiled in one place, and I knew I had to do something with it. So in the midst of my grief over the loss of my fertility, and just as the battle began to accomplish my goal of having another child, I decided to write this book. Fortunately, a week after I signed the contract, I got the good news—I was pregnant! So, while compiling all the information you have in your hands, organizing it, and putting it down in print, a little life grew inside me, and on occasion reminded me with a swift kick why I decided to put all my other professional endeavors on hold and create this resource for women.

This is the book I went looking for, and couldn't find. I wanted to know everything there is to know about the biological clock, and why mine decided to quit so suddenly and so completely. What you are about to read is what I discovered over three years of my struggle, as well as more than six months of intense research and writing. In addition to a comprehensive review of medical literature and personal experiences, however, you will find plenty of practical advice. I grew tired of reading article after article that predicted doom and gloom for professional single women in their 30s and 40s. I knew, and continue to believe, that much of the doom and gloom—that is, childlessness—results from lack of knowledge. The fact is, women need to know much more about their reproductive life span, and they need to know what they can *do* about getting the most out of it.

Here's the way I see it: Millions of you are not trying to get pregnant, so you have no way to know whether you would be having trouble or not, and you have no idea that, at the very least, you can check your fertility with a simple blood test. Many of you have boyfriends and are talking about getting engaged, married, and having children, and some of you are already married, but waiting for one reason or another to start your families. Am I talking about you? Do you know someone like this? Don't wait; there are lots of things you can do: take an FSH test; check your cycle; use birth control pills; make an appointment with a reproductive endocrinologist; freeze your eggs or embryos if you're married—the list goes on. Be proactive with your clock—don't let it wind down while you aren't looking!

My struggle is over now, but knowing that this book, and its tremendous amount of practical information now exists for others, is incredibly rewarding. In fact, all my action has given birth to both a beautiful daughter and a much needed resource on one of the most important aspects of a woman's health: her biological clock.

This, of course, was an accident of circumstance. I came face to face with my useless clock almost exactly one year after my son was born. Little did I know it had stopped, and I would have no choice but to come to think of him as my miracle child. In fact, I often say, "He was my last good egg!" Four and a half years later, my second miracle child was born. Though as you read along, you will realize that she was infinitely more work to conceive—infertility treatments, disappointments, several miscarriages, weekly counseling sessions, insurance battles, five egg-donor searches, attorney consultations, support groups, biweekly acupuncture, countless doctors' appointments, and other hitches and roadblocks to overcome before casting my eyes on the child that has made our lives complete. Now that she is here, yes, she was worth every tear and last ounce of energy I managed to summon.

Although I have longed for this day, I also hope that what you will find in the following pages will help you avoid a similar struggle. At the very least, you will know everything there is to know about your biological clock, and that is a major step toward gaining control over your reproductive future. I wish you all the best.

Take a Look at Your Biological Clock

1.

Hormones Can Tell What Time It Is

I got the results of my first FSH test *in the mail*. In fact, the tone of the letter was hauntingly unassuming:

Dear Ms. Birrittieri,

Just a note to let you know the results of your blood work. Your blood type is O positive and you are immune to German measles. Your levels of thyroid hormone, prolactin, and estrogen were normal.

Next paragraph:

The FSH level is elevated at 19.6 (we like to see values under 10). This is strongly suggestive of impaired ovarian reserve....

My reaction? "Hmmm, that last part doesn't sound so good. What's *FSH*, and what on earth could *impaired ovarian reserve* mean?" I had no idea, but I got a skin-crawling, creepy sensation as I read it over and over and over again. I was scared to death. A few weeks later, I summoned the courage to do an online search for both terms. What I found hurt, shocked, and infuriated me.

FSH is follicle-stimulating hormone, and levels in blood serum indicate adequate or poor ovarian reserve. The bottom line (and it took all of about two minutes online for me to figure this out): if you have higher levels of FSH, you are basically running short on eggs! I couldn't believe it! I just had a baby, how could I be running low on eggs? It took awhile for the information to sink in. Although I was a biology major, science teacher, and became a journalist who regularly reported on health and medicine, the idea that I was one day going to *run out of eggs* somehow escaped me. The realization was difficult to face, especially now—I had just accomplished one of my lifelong goals: motherhood. This sudden revelation couldn't have hit at a worse time. My naturally conceived son was barely walking, my mommy hormones were at their peak, and I wanted one more child— just *one* more!

While the thought of my dwindling supply of tiny eggs crept into my every thought, I also felt a plume of smoke blasting out each ear—I was mad, really mad. For the previous decade, I was a career woman, yes, but after a certain point, not necessarily by choice. I always wanted a profession *and* children, and therefore I was keenly aware of that increasingly clamorous "ticktock" of my biological clock. I worried, but tried not to let it overwhelm me. After all, for most of my 30s I was single, with no long-term mate prospects in sight. But there I was, 41, married, with a 1-year-old adorable baby boy, looking at this FSH result and thinking, *WHAT? There is a test that can tell you what time it is on your biological clock? I've been wondering that for years; worrying I might run out of time, and now you tell me I'm probably past the deadline—all from a simple blood test?*

I can't even express how upset I was that nobody told me about this test. During my six-week follow-up visit with my obstetrician following the birth of my son, I remember discussing the fact that I wanted another child, and she said, "Try to be pregnant within a year." Good advice, but what about checking my FSH level immediately to see if a year would be too late? I never heard that. However, as soon as I walked into an infertility clinic, it was ordered without any fanfare, or explanation, right alongside my blood type.

After learning the devastating news, the idea that it was delivered via snail mail just added salt to the open wound. I never went back to that clinic. Instead, I did some homework and quickly found a top-notch, thorough, and caring reproductive endocrinologist. I immediately bombarded him with questions as only a reporter could.

The first question: "Why don't more people know about this test?" His response went something like this: most obstetrician-gynecologists don't bother with it, either because they're too busy with other things like delivering babies, or they don't know enough about it as a fertility gauge to even consider offering it, or both. Upon further informal discussions with doctors and patients, it seems they are also reluctant to ask about a woman's plans to have children, fearing treading too far into personal territory. Primary care, or family doctors, shy away from such conversations as well, and might order an FSH test only if an older woman is having obvious symptoms of menopause. Hence, younger women, in their 30s and early 40s, tend to learn about this test only if they are having difficulty getting pregnant, and seek a specialist at an infertility clinic.

Once I realized countless women are missing this critical information, I decided it was time for a change; writing this book would become the first step.

Tissues Are a Must
When Giving the High FSH Talk

Dr. Pat McShane runs a successful clinic northwest of Boston. The morning I visited with her, she had already given the "high FSH" talk *three* times—to a 35-year-old, a 36-year-old, and a 41-year-old. "It's devastating news to be giving to somebody. The look of surprise and anguish that I see is heart wrenching. You really want to leap across the desk and hug these poor people because you know what a difficult road they will be heading down if they choose treatment—many of them will succeed but many others will not. So, it's very unpleasant and sad for people. I always keep a box of tissues nearby."

Often many of these patients have been going to the same gynecologists or obstetricians for years. Even if they ask about having children, or another child, they are often reassured rather than given medical information related to fertility, or offered an FSH test. Such was the case with Kathy, the mother of one of my son's preschool friends who has been trying for two years to have a second child. As soon she sought out an infertility clinic, she got the high FSH talk, and was furious. "I had a baby at 36 and now four years later, I'm told

I have a 2-percent chance using the best technology available. I have done several treatment cycles with no success. I am angry and heartbroken."

She had been going to the same OB-GYN for a decade and boldly confronted her doctor after receiving the devastating news. "I said, 'I've been coming here for 10 years, why didn't you say anything?' She replied, 'It's not my place to talk about having babies, some people take it the wrong way—we are not in the business of steering people in certain directions.'"

Kathy says that excuse was unacceptable. "Her answer made me even more angry, because it is a doctor's job to provide medical information. And that's what I needed: medical information—before I started having trouble—not medical information once I had to walk into an infertility clinic. Gynecologists have no trouble talking about contraception, so they shouldn't have any trouble talking about the time frame for children. This is educating women about their bodies; it's not prying, and it shouldn't have to be done inside infertility clinics when, by that time, it's usually too late."

Women, including you and your girlfriends, need to know that there is a way to get a peek at the time on your clock: the FSH blood test. It isn't a crystal clear observation, but it is as good as it gets for a simple blood test. Across this country, every day there are hundreds if not thousands of women taking FSH tests *after* having problems for one, two, or three or more years. Infertility specialists use it routinely to determine what their problems likely are. These doctors are rarely wrong if the woman is 35 or over and the FSH is elevated. Though a 35-, 38-, or 40-year-old woman may have perfectly regular periods, even a slightly elevated FSH test tells them she is probably in the early stages of fertility decline. It doesn't mean she can't get pregnant, it simply means the chances are dropping rapidly, and depending on the FSH level and her age, her odds may be next to nothing, even with the best technology available.

Do you see a problem here? Women often end up taking this test past the point of little or no return. Therefore, some reproductive endocrinologists believe it's high time other doctors, internists, family physicians, and especially OB-GYNs start offering it as part of routine care for women. McShane says it should be offered to all women in their mid-30s as a baseline. "Women over 35 should have an

FSH level checked by their OB-GYN. Why not be armed with the knowledge? It's not going to guarantee that you are going to be okay, but if you are not okay, that's important to know." Many fertility specialists agree women should have access to, or at least more information about, the FSH and other ovarian reserve tests, still others disagree for reasons I will highlight later.

Follicle-Stimulating Hormone

Follicle-stimulating hormone does exactly what its name implies, it stimulates follicles. Follicles are the cellular sacs in which individual eggs mature. During each cycle, one of these eggs will burst from the follicle, in the process called ovulation, and meet it's fate one way or another as it travels down the fallopian tube. The follicle tissue itself becomes what's called the corpus luteum, which goes on to produce more pregnancy-related hormones if that egg meets up with a sperm, is fertilized, and results in a viable pregnancy. So it is FSH that drives the system each month. This important hormone recruits several follicles inside the ovary, their eggs will begin to mature, and one will eventually go on to ovulation.

FSH is part of the hormonal messaging system that operates between your brain and your ovaries each month. The process kicks off with another hormone called gonadotropin-releasing hormone (GnRH) that is produced by the brain's hypothalamus. (FSH is one kind of gonadotropin hormone.) Once GnRH enters the system, it tells the pituitary gland to start releasing FSH. This hormone then signals the ovaries to throw the switch and wake up some long dormant egg-containing follicles and start their engines.

In a woman who is 20-something, these eggs roll out of their sleepy state easily, and their engines start revving with out much trouble. In a woman who is 30-something, or better yet, in her early 40s, FSH has a harder time rousting up a new crew of follicles every month, and the eggs inside need a lot more coaxing to get their engines started. Think of the younger ovaries as full of follicles and eggs that are akin to shiny new race cars; and the older ovaries containing follicles that are more like a small collection of rare classic Fords.

Using this analogy, the FSH molecules are like people recruiting cars and drivers for a major race. Now, if a bunch of Edsels show up for a Nascar event, it's obvious that something is wrong! This is just

21

like the pituitary receiving the news that there is not enough of the right kind of eggs, so it starts pumping out *more* FSH; these molecules rush to the ovaries to try to roust more eggs. The harder it is to recruit follicles for any given cycle, the more the pituitary produces FSH, and the higher the concentrations of FSH in the blood.

As the reproductive clock ticks closer and closer to the point where fertility begins a steep downward slide, FSH begins to rise. This very early, slow, yet incremental increase can be detected in the blood, and tells clinicians that your ovaries are not as responsive as they once were because the number of follicles is beginning to decline. The standard FSH blood test has routinely shown that the higher the FSH levels, the lower the chances for a viable pregnancy with treatment, even with the most aggressive technology.

History of FSH Testing

The early precursor to today's FSH blood test was an interesting procedure involving, of all things, rats. In its time, this test was a revolutionary breakthrough that allowed obstetricians and gynecologists dealing with infertility issues to determine whether difficulties getting pregnant might be attributable to premature menopause. In fact, this test was as high tech as you could get back in 1939, when the first department of reproductive medicine was created in the United States. The woman who was appointed to head the department at Johns Hopkins, Dr. Georgeanna Jones, of the now famous Jones Institute for Reproductive Medicine in Norfolk, Virginia, happened to be one of the few FSH experts at that time, and the rat test was one of the first done in her new department of reproductive medicine more than 65 years ago. (Georgeanna and her husband, Dr. Howard Jones Jr., were responsible for the first IVF [in vitro fertilization] baby born in the United States.)

At that time, FSH was extracted from a woman's urine rather than her blood. Doctors would purify the FSH from the urine sample as best they could and inject it into the tail vein of a rat. The extra FSH in the rat causes the rat's uterus and ovaries to enlarge. *Three days later*, the rat would undergo a hysterectomy and doctors would simply weigh the organs. The weight would be described in so many "rat units." These rat units told the physician whether his patient's FSH was elevated to the point of menopause. Dr. Howard Jones says the test was primitive but "it would be very important for a

32-year-old who came in and hadn't had a period for two years. You would do the urine test and find out if she had menopausal levels of FSH, and was in premature menopause. It was very useful to us."

FSH Fertility Drug Development

While doctors refined the testing to detect their patients' FSH levels, scientists in hot pursuit of FSH collected it any way they could to develop fertility drugs. In the beginning, they extracted it from animals—horses, pigs, and primates. They also isolated FSH from the logical human source, the pituitary gland; however, none of these routes produced the quality nor the quantity in demand—a demand which was expected to rise.

However, in the late 1940s scientists working for the Italian company Serono showed that FSH and other proteins extracted from the *urine* of menopausal women induced eggs to grow in the ovaries of rats. This finding eventually established the first promising follicle stimulating medication for women, Pergonal. Vice president of clinical development at Serono, Louis O'Dea says FSH was a target for drug development before anyone knew exactly what it was. "Generally, when researchers are able to identify that something is present, they start immediately looking for ways to extract it and use it as a drug. The problem was isolating it in a pure enough form."

Encouraged by it's success, Serono pressed on, committing to producing the drug on a large scale. It was no easy task to collect urine from post-menopausal women, extract the FSH, and mass-produce the injectable drug. This first of its kind pharmaceutical endeavor took place in Italy, where Serono enlisted the services of a tremendously generous group of women. According to O'Dea, "It was really similar to blood donation in the sense that it was done altruistically, by all of the volunteers. They were the little old grandmothers in the small villages in the small towns in Italy, and folklore has it that elderly Roman Catholic nuns were also involved. The women were healthy older women, who on a daily basis donated [urine]. A small van came through the village and picked up and dropped off the bottles. It was really a simple system."

Over the ensuing years it became difficult to constantly replenish the supplies of urine for manufacturing; by 1985 approximately 6,600 gallons of urine were needed *every day* to meet the demand for Serono's

23

fertility products. It wasn't long before the company turned to bio-technology to artificially synthesize pure FSH through recombinant DNA technology. Once this was accomplished, the postmenopausal women were off the hook. Today Serono is the leading manufacturer of recombinant FSH, sold as Gonal-F.

Almost as soon as this new drug became available, doctors had patients who wanted to use it. Long before the first successful in vitro fertilization (IVF) procedure, physicians prescribed these medications to women simply to stimulate the growth of their follicles and induce ovulation so couples could have a better chance of achieving a pregnancy on their own. During this time, doctors used the FSH test to help determine if women were close to menopause as an indication of whether this medication might work, and, once treatment was underway, to monitor whether the drug was having any effect on hormone levels. It wasn't until a decade *after* the first in vitro baby was born that scientists tried using the FSH test in the context of *fertility potential* and treatment outcome, rather than simply as a crude measurement to detect premature menopause.

First FSH Test to Predict Treatment Response

Dr. Georgeanna Jones was again at the cutting edge of this technology. In a landmark study published in 1988, she, along with several others at the Jones Institute for Reproductive Medicine, including Dr. Zev Rosenwaks (now the director of the Center for Reproductive Medicine and Infertility at Cornell University's Weill Medical College), were first to establish the FSH blood test as an indicator of how a particular woman might respond while undergoing IVF treatment. The paper showed for the first time that checking a woman's FSH level on *day three* of her menstrual cycle could help predict how well her ovaries would respond to FSH medications, and ultimately what her chances would be of becoming pregnant via IVF. Researchers found that women with the highest FSH levels had the poorest response and were the least likely to get pregnant.

Further research has focused on the predictive value of the FSH level, as well as other tests that provide a peek at the biological clock.

All of these tests came about during the explosion in IVF. The reason for this is simple: doctors wanted a way to determine whether it was useful for a woman to undergo IVF before she actually did.

This highly technical procedure is very expensive and devastating when it does not work.

It turns out that IVF provided the perfect subjects for understanding how to predict fertility potential. With IVF, doctors know precisely how many eggs have responded to the FSH drugs, how many of them fertilized, and whether or not they were capable of creating a viable pregnancy. Hence, once the blood test is taken, doctors can later accurately measure whether the levels mean anything. This kind of research continues today and has revealed unprecedented information about the biological clock. Hormonal tests are in use across the country inside reproductive medicine clinics, and although they aren't perfect, they are the best that medicine can offer to women who are already having trouble conceiving. Many believe these tests can also help other women gauge their clocks *before* it's too late.

Today's Day Three FSH Test

The "day three FSH test" is the gold standard for testing for ovarian reserve at all reproductive medicine clinics. A reproductive endocrinologist (RE) will order the test for any woman over 35 who simply walks in the door. Depending on the patient's history, including whether she smokes and her mother's age at menopause, the same RE might order it for a woman well below age 35. The idea is to rule out the most common problem first.

How Do I Take an FSH Test?

Let's make one thing perfectly clear: you don't have to be having problems to take an FSH test; you don't even have to be trying to get pregnant! This is a blood test you have done on the third day of your menstrual cycle. You simply count the first day of a full flow as day one. What if you start flowing at night? Clinics say if you start flowing after 6 p.m., the next day is day one. As you can imagine, the timing can be a bit daunting. Your day three could fall on a weekend, a business trip, or Thanksgiving. This is why reproductive medicine clinics have hours on weekends and holidays. However, you can have the test whenever you need it. You simply get a blood test order from your doctor and on your day three, bring it to the nearest hospital to have your blood drawn. Whether it's your birthday, Easter Sunday, or

Hanukkah, you can get the job done as long as you have the written order from your doctor.

There are two routes to requesting that written order. You can simply go to a reproductive medicine clinic, or you can ask your OB-GYN or primary care doctor. If you live near a major city or know of a reproductive medicine clinic in your vicinity, that would be the best option. Here's why: Fertility experts know how the FSH test is used to detect the first signs of decreased fertility due to age. Anybody can tell you that an FSH of 50 is in the menopausal range, but a fertility specialist is best trained to explain to you what an FSH of 12 means.

The next best thing is to make an appointment with your OB-GYN or primary care doctor, whichever you feel most comfortable asking, and tell him or her you want the test done. Don't be surprised if she thinks you are nuts. Most family doctors and gynecologists use the FSH test as a menopause test, so if you are not pushing 50, she might question you. Tell her it's an FSH test to check in on your fertility long before menopause. If she remains resistant, explain what you know about the test, and ask for help. If that doesn't work, try another doctor.

Once you get your lab order, ask the doctor to bill your insurance company as part of a routine visit. Often you'll be able to go back to the lab connected to the doctor's office if your day three falls on a weekday. However, if your day three falls on a weekend or holiday, ask her where she might suggest you go. Sometimes even doctors' office-building labs have some limited weekend hours. Or you can do a little homework, make a few phone calls, to find out the closest lab that draws blood on a weekend. That's usually a local emergency room, but there may also be a walk-in clinic in your area.

One more thing: If you are taking a birth control pill, you will have to go off the prescription to do this test. The pill contains estrogen, which as you will see later, inhibits FSH. So if you don't stop the pill for the cycle prior to the test, the results will be invalid. The estrogen in the pill will mask the true level of FSH. So, as soon as you decide to do this test, plan to remain off the pill for one month, then have your blood drawn on day three of your next *natural* period. Afterward, you can start back on your pill according to the prescription instructions.

Cover Your Assay!

There are two basic types of assays laboratories use to detect FSH in the blood. One type employs radioactive isotopes that attach onto the FSH molecules, and the other type doesn't. Instead, this type uses antibodies, which attract and bind the FSH molecules. The radioactive isotope assay (RIA) is the older method, and arguably the most sensitive and accurate, but also the most time consuming and unwieldy because it requires the use of radioactive particles.

If you are going to a fertility clinic to do your FSH testing, you may not have to worry about "covering your assay" as much, but if you are going to a primary care or OB-GYN doctor, you should understand these two methods for determining your FSH level. The reason is important: the two types of assays will produce different FSH counts, and you and your doctor have to be able to interpret the results correctly. Again, this is a no-brainer if you are perimenopausal, or menopausal, because the levels will be quite high, but if you want a peek at the biological clock when it's either very much intact, or just on the verge of slowing down, knowing the type of assay that is being used is critical.

That said, if you are going to a lab unconnected to an infertility clinic, most likely you won't be receiving the RIA, but it is imperative you ask to make sure. Also, sometimes the blood sample will be sent off to a contracted company to perform the test, so get the name of the laboratory where your blood will be sent, and find out if they will be using an RIA or a standard immunoassay that uses the antibody method. This way you will have a better understanding as soon as you see the results, rather than waiting and wondering if your doctor got it right. Again, the lab will likely be using the newer, more efficient, often very automated "immunoassay" using antibodies rather than the RIA, but you want to be sure.

The basic difference is this: because the RIA is more sensitive, it picks up more of the FSH molecules, therefore, it gives you a higher reading overall. So in clinics that still use the RIA, the extreme danger zone starts at 20 units, whereas in clinics that use the antibody test, doctors will deliver really bad news when the results are much lower. How much lower? In general, when the standard antibody test shows a level between 10 and 15 units, this implies your clock is nearly stopped, your fertility is rapidly declining, and you should take action immediately. That could mean anything from trying to get pregnant right away, including getting into treatment as soon as possible, or if you're single, it could mean even finding a sperm donor and either trying for a pregnancy right away, with or with out medical intervention, or doing IVF so you can freeze embryos until you are ready for a child. Though the IVF route can be pricey, these are real options for single women, and few realize they are available.

Any FSH level over 15 units means you have hit the rapid drop in fertility, there's no going back, and your chances even with treatment are 5 percent or less. My *first* FSH was 19.6 a year after my son was born. This decline can happen rapidly regardless of when you had your last naturally conceived child. After a few more FSH tests, my doctor informed me that given my age and FSH levels, my chances were probably *1* percent, and if I'm lucky, maybe 5 percent.

All women think they are going to hit the jackpot, but remember, on average, this means 95 out of 100 women who try IVF will not be successful. I had a brief talk with myself and decided I did not feel that lucky. I was never a gambler anyway, even with much higher odds, so we decided against IVF and tried on our own a little longer. We did the sensible thing and put our financial resources toward other options just in case our "natural" cycles didn't work out. (More on this story in Chapter 5.)

Typical results with the immunoassay show levels under 10 are considered good, but if they're hovering around 10, your ovaries could be signaling the very early, initial decline in fertility. If you are under 35 years old and in the FSH range of 3 to 7, you are probably fine.

If you happen upon a clinic or lab using the RIA, these levels are pushed up a bit. Levels that are at 20 and above mean you have probably hit the rapid decline and chances of a good outcome in treatment are in the 5-percent range. The closer to 20, the lower your chances. Anything in the 10 to 15 range indicates you are likely okay. Generally, the clinic can best explain your results. Doctors will have specific success rates based on FSH levels, and can offer you the best advice given your particular result.

FSH Pitfalls and Limitations

Although the day three FSH test is a standard test used by fertility experts, it is generally one of the first diagnostic tests given to a new infertility patient, and treatment options are provided based on its results, it does have limitations. In fact, the fertility experts who use this test day in and day out will be the first to tell you this test is a guide, not an absolute.

Most research on the day three FSH test shows this test is an indicator of the *quantity*, not necessarily the *quality* of your eggs. So it appears that in younger women (early to mid-30s) even if the level is over 10, and ovarian reserve appears to be on the slide, there may be a fairly good ratio of good eggs versus bad. So in a treatment setting, doctors might advise women younger than 40 to try IVF; however, they may not go so far as to say they can wait a year or two to start a family. *Any elevated FSH level is an indication that your clock is working harder to stay up to speed.*

Elevated FSH levels in women in their late 30s and early 40s correlate with higher miscarriage rates and poor pregnancy rates, indicating that a drop in *quality* due to age has caught up to the lack of quantity. The current thinking among the experts is that if you have an elevated FSH and you are under 40, all is not lost, and if you are over 40, all could be lost. Notice there is no absolute. The only time a fertility expert will give you an absolute is when you are menopausal, and the FSH levels remain very high after repeated tests. The point is, everyone knows women can and do get pregnant with elevated FSH, but they are the lottery winners. For every one or two of them, there are a hundred others who bought and paid dearly for the ticket, but lost the prize.

Another important caveat to the FSH test is the fact that FSH levels fluctuate from cycle to cycle. For this reason you shouldn't depend on the results of one FSH test. You could have an FSH level of 14 on one test, come back in three months and retest to find it at 7 this time, but three months after that, it might be at 15.5. Think of a company's rising annual stock chart. One month the stock is up, the next it's down, but the overall trend is always upward. This is good news for the stockowner, bad news for women monitoring their biological clocks. Also, research indicates that your fertility is only as good as your worst or highest FSH level. Reproductive endocrinologists always use the *worst* result as their guide for treatment.

The fact of the matter is, even if you have a low FSH level, you know eventually it will begin to climb; there's nothing you can do to control it, and when it begins its ascent, you know your fertility is waning. At this point, there is no time to waste if you want to put what ever time you have left toward having a child. You can use this test to monitor your clock. Don't hesitate, even though you can't control this process, you can at least check in on it from time to time.

One more important note about interpreting the results. If you go to your family doctor or OB-GYN, it is important to use the values here as a guide to your fertility. (You can also find similar basic information on FSH test results online and through various infertility organizations.) The companies that manufacture immunoassay kits also provide the doctor with information on what their normal ranges are. The critical word here is *normal*. The booklet guide for one popular automated test says for a day three FSH, a normal result would be anywhere from 3 to 14.4. The problem is, the group of women that generated these guidelines ranged in age from 16 to 44 years old. Of course an FSH of 14.4 is *normal* for a 44-year-old! However, it doesn't mean you will be able to have a child. On the contrary, this is not a good result if you are hoping to have children. So make sure you discuss your result thoroughly with your doctor. He or she may say, "Oh, your result is *normal*," when in fact, it may be normal, but just awful for baby-making. If there is any question in your mind, consult a reproductive endocrinologist for the best advice on your reproductive clock and what your options may be. Don't be surprised if he or she asks you to do another FSH test on your next cycle. Remember, these tests are a glimpse into the clock, so the more you look over a period of time, the clearer the picture becomes.

Use It or Lose It

It's high time the FSH test is offered to women starting at age 35, especially if they are considering having a child. (It's been available and put to great use in reproductive medicine for nearly 20 years!) Also, more family doctors, obstetricians, and gynecologists should add it to their arsenal of tests to help empower women to make better, more informed (and healthier) choices in life. Had I known about this test when I gave birth at 40, I would have taken it as soon as I started my period again. I'm sure I was already in the danger zone, and would have been able to make an informed decision as to whether I wanted to risk waiting or try for another baby right away. Instead, I figured I was fertile because I just had a baby, so I didn't take immediate action. One year later, there was to be no baby. This lack of information put me through a hell that I hope you never experience. Even if it is bad news, knowing is better than not knowing when it comes to your fertility.

However, many doctors, including reproductive endocrinologists, will say the FSH test is not worth using as a preventative measure. The majority says it's because it doesn't predict how much time you have left. Others say it's not reliable because it fluctuates and, therefore, is unnecessary for women who aren't having trouble getting pregnant because it may give them a false sense of security. Still others argue it only means something if the level is elevated. As an informed patient, and someone who sees tremendous value in using the test as a way to prevent infertility, these arguments don't make sense. Any accurate information a woman receives via an FSH test is better than no information, if she is concerned about her biological clock.

Often the test doesn't even cross the minds of obstetricians and gynecologists. Women see these physicians annually and they ought to talk about all aspects of their reproductive health. Countless women undergo IVF, donor egg, and sometimes both procedures only because their gynecologists never asked about their plans for having children and didn't consider offering an FSH test to check for signs of trouble. Many obstetricians can also be unconcerned about fertility. But women who already have a child are going to lose their infertility too. Mothers need to be just as aware because they may want more children. If doctors understood the physical and emotional toll infertility and its treatment take on women, couples, and families, they would see this as a burning women's health issue. Unfortunately, they rarely encounter the agony women suffer, because the tears are shed inside reproductive medicine clinics, not their offices.

Take Action Sooner Rather Than Later

Why should fertility be off-limits, and contraception so easy to talk about? Women need fertility information to learn about their reproductive clock even in a short visit for an annual Pap smear or a follow-up visit after a birth.

At the moment, few women realize the simple FSH test exists, and those who do often wait too long to utilize it. Case in point, Lisa, a 40-year-old executive, walked into one of Boston's most popular reproductive medicine clinics and asked for a fertility workup. She is single and wants to decide whether she should try to have a baby using a sperm donor. She obviously wants children, but for one reason or another never met Mr. Right. But she is *40*. Somewhere along the way, she, along with millions of other women, missed the fact that fertility starts to decline in the late 20s, and on average right around 40, it basically falls off a cliff. She has the right idea, and is obviously informed enough to know where she can go to find out what time it is, but she may have taken action too late.

Caution: Over-the-Counter Hormone Tests

Back in 2001, the Food and Drug Administration (FDA) approved the first home test that detects FSH in the urine. These tests are now marketed to women 35 and over via the Internet, and in your local pharmacies as home "menopause" monitors, or tests. They all measure FSH levels in the urine, but they measure relatively high amounts. That is, in order to get a positive result, your FSH must be at a level of 25, well into the perimenopausal stage. Most manufacturers say the test is not a fertility test and shouldn't be used as such. Some companies, however, claim their tests can be used periodically to gauge whether women have entered perimenopause and are approaching the end of fertility. While that may be true, by the time you get a positive result on the test, you can certainly expect to have tremendous difficulty achieving pregnancy, and may not be able to have a child at all.

So, unless you are *hoping* to reach the infertile part of your life, and are already experiencing perimenopausal symptoms such as night sweats and hot flashes, irregular periods, and insomnia, these tests are not recommended. Don't waste your money or your time; it is best to seek out a physician, preferably at a reproductive medicine clinic, to help you take a look at your biological clock. These home FSH tests can only tell when your clock has taken a lickin' and is hardly tickin'.

Other Hormone Tests to Check Your Clock

Reproductive endocrinologists use a battery of other "ovarian function" or "ovarian reserve" tests to help them advise patients on treatment options and their various success rates. These too can be used in the context of prevention, though they rarely are. These tests, like the FSH test, were developed specifically to help assess age-related infertility for women already having difficulties. All the research has been done in women undergoing treatment for infertility. However, few reproductive experts would dispute that the patients they were designed to help are those most likely experiencing age-related infertility. Therefore, it seems to me they can help clear the view of your clock beforehand as well.

These are more sophisticated tests and should be interpreted in conjunction with the FSH level. Depending on how comfortable your OB-GYN is with this kind of testing, you may be able to do both the Estradiol and Clomid Challenge Tests with him or her; however, the others should be overseen by a board certified reproductive endocrinologist for the most accurate fertility assessment possible.

Estradiol (E2)

Estradiol, or *E2* for short, is estrogen. The level of E2 in your blood is best taken at the same time as your day three FSH test (taken on days two, three, or four). This can help detect ovarian decline because it can further clarify whether a low day three FSH result is accurate. When fertility is normal, both the FSH level and the E2 level should be low. Exactly what a low, or acceptable, level for E2 is remains debatable. Normal ranges for day three are roughly 25 to 75. Generally a day three E2 level greater than 75 or 80 is considered abnormally high. If the corresponding FSH level is low, then this raises a red flag. It means that the elevated estrogen could be suppressing FSH, resulting in an artificially low result. Which could mean your excellent FSH news may not be accurate. Checking the E2 level alongside your FSH is a good idea, just in case your results fall into this category. If they do, the Clomid Challenge Test, discussed next, is generally recommended.

If your estrogen levels are at the other end of the spectrum, that is, below 25 or 30, this could signal a problem due to excessive exercise and/or low percentage of body fat, which causes estrogen levels to drop—not a good situation for your fertility (see Chapter 4). Low estrogen may also signal that you are on your way to an early menopause if your FSH levels are also very high. If your results show any of these conditions, you should consult a reproductive endocrinologist for further testing and/or treatment.

The Clomid Challenge Test

Clomiphene citrate (also known as *Clomid*) is a synthetic drug and is the most commonly prescribed fertility medication. It stimulates the hypothalamus to produce a hormone that prompts the pituitary to release more FSH. Increasing your FSH, as you know, pushes your ovaries to produce more eggs. Even before they first published work on the day three FSH test, the previously mentioned Norfolk Virginia researchers came up with the idea for using Clomid alongside FSH testing for ovarian reserve. In 1987 they gave this test to a group of 51 women ages 35 or over with unexplained infertility—and fertility clinics have been using this Clomiphene citrate challenge test (CCCT) ever since.

The test consists of a day three FSH blood test followed by a regimen of 100 mg of Clomid taken orally on day five through day nine of the cycle, and then repeating the FSH test on day 10. E2 measurements are generally taken on these days as well. If your day three FSH is in the normal range, and everything is fine, the Clomid will have no effect, and your day 10 FSH level will also be low, or perhaps even lower than your day three level. If your day 10 level is elevated at all, this is indicative of a slowing clock, or to use the vernacular, "diminished ovarian reserve."

Newer Tests Best Done at a Reproductive Medicine Clinic

Clinicians and researchers are working on other more precise methods of evaluating the reproductive clock. So far they haven't found any one test that can accurately predict how much time a woman has left to have children, or if she's already considering treatment, whether she can become pregnant. The following tests, however, show promise.

Inhibin B

Evidence suggests that a relatively newly discovered hormone called *inhibin B* can give you a look at the biological clock. This research claims testing levels of inhibin B on day three of your menstrual cycle can be even more accurate than the FSH level. Some believe that because inhibin B is produced by the follicles that are beginning to develop in the ovaries (also called antral follicles), it is an *earlier* marker for ovaries that are running out of eggs. Therefore, if you are running out of eggs, the fewer follicles developing for each cycle, the less inhibin B. Researchers also think this reduced inhibin B level allows FSH to rise—a necessity in order to recruit at least one dominant follicle for ovulation from the ever-disappearing pool of eggs. One study indeed showed that low inhibin B level on day three correlates with a decreased response to fertility medication, fewer eggs retrieved, and lower pregnancy rate in women undergoing IVF.

Another study compared FSH levels and inhibin levels and concluded inhibin B was a better predictor of pregnancy rate than FSH. The study found women with good FSH levels and poor inhibin B levels had a pregnancy rate of only 4 percent; women with poor FSH levels and good inhibin B levels had a pregnancy rate of 17.6 percent; and women with both good FSH and good inhibin B levels had the best chance of pregnancy at 36.9 percent. In this study, an adequate inhibin B level was anything *over* 45, and a good FSH level was a level of 10 or *under*.

The assays for the inhibin B test are also highly variable, and because it is not routine, results should be reviewed by an experienced fertility expert well versed in ovarian reserve testing. But from the current evidence, it appears this test can wipe a little more grit off the face of your clock, for an even better look.

Anti-Mullerian Hormone

Anti-Mullerian hormone (AMH) is also known as Mullerian-inhibiting substance (MIS). Testing for blood levels of this hormone is the newest, and to some experts the most promising, of the clock screening tests. Because research is just beginning, however, it is unlikely you will have access to it in the near future. Still, given the excitement about the preliminary research, it is important to know it exists, and may one day become the screening test of choice for fertility potential.

This hormone is secreted by very early ovarian follicles, even *before* they start their initial growth spurt toward ovulation. Researchers believe that the level of anti-Mullerian hormone circulating in the blood is a good indication of the *total* number of viable eggs within the ovary. All the other markers discussed so far are indirect markers of the number of follicles that are already undergoing stimulation by FSH (either naturally or via fertility drugs). AMH is produced by all the follicles sitting in the back of the egg assembly line; hence, the more AMH detected, the more eggs in your basket, so to speak.

Size, Volume, and Antral Follicle Count

Though most fertility experts have focused on hormonal markers to provide a look at what time it is on the reproductive clock, another method is also gaining attention. It's a relatively low-tech procedure that involves simply taking a look at the ovaries—checking their size, determining their volume, and literally counting the number of small developing follicles that can be seen. All this is done with an ultrasound probe that is inserted into the vagina (transvaginal ultrasound) to get a close-up look at the ovaries.

Women's ovaries are smaller following menopause than they are prior to the change in life. However, a recent study reveals more precisely when this shrinkage occurs. Researchers at the University of Kentucky Medical Center studied the annual ultrasounds of nearly 14,000 women from ages 25 to 91 over several years as part of an ovarian cancer screening program. The data shows the total volume of the ovaries in women under 30 on average was 6.6 cm^3 (cubic centimeters); with volume decreasing steadily with an average of just 2.1 cm^3 in women ages 60 to 69. Interestingly, this study also found that the volume of the ovaries had no bearing on weight, but was greater in tall women than in short women.

Ovarian volume has also been shown to be a fairly good indicator of outcome in fertility treatment, especially IVF. One study concluded that women with an ovarian volume of less than 3 cm^3 produced fewer follicles and had much lower chance of a successful outcome than those with larger ovaries.

More recently, rather than outright measuring the ovaries, researchers are counting the observable tiny *antral* follicles within them. Several studies have shown antral follicle count (AFC) can predict ovarian aging and potential pregnancy success with treatment. Some clinics do an antral follicle count as part of their diagnostic workup, and some perform the procedure to help determine the best protocol for treatment. Either way, it appears that fertility experts are becoming increasingly interested in counting the small follicles that are always bubbling up from the reserve of resting primordial follicles inside the ovaries.

Doctors believe, and some research has shown, that the number of these activated follicles is a snapshot of the amount remaining in the ovaries. In other words, the more follicles that awaken, the more there are still hibernating back in the den. As a woman ages, the antral follicle count appears to drop according to the number of eggs or follicles the menstrual cycle has to draw from. One early study, which focused on normal women with proven fertility, shows that up to age 37 the number of follicles declined by a rate of 4.8 percent per year, but after that, it dropped quickly to nearly 12 percent.

Unfortunately, like the other tests described here, there is still no way to accurately predict how much time remains on *your* biological clock. However, given that the antral follicle count and other ovarian reserve tests are extremely valuable to those already seeking to become pregnant, they can also be used to give you an indication of your current fertility status. Researchers in the field of reproductive medicine are working toward tests that can accurately predict how much time a woman has to put her fertility to use. This research hopes to answer the question many women ask as they listen to that annoying ticktock, "What time is it?"

Marcelle Cedars, M.D., director of the Division of Reproductive Endocrinology at the University of California, San Francisco, hopes to give women a precise method to determine how much time they have to become mothers. "We want to study a large population of women of differing ethnicities to evaluate the rate of antral follicle change, and then also compare it with a genetic factor." Cedars plans to establish some guidelines on the rates of egg loss in normal women, so women can discern how quickly they are losing eggs, and therefore how soon they should start their families. She says this kind of research has never been more important. "The difference is, 20 years ago, a woman at 39 might be concerned because she is having trouble conceiving her third or fourth child, whereas now she is really in dire straits, because she is having difficulty trying for her *first* child."

Unfortunately, like most research concerning reproductive medicine, funding is extremely competitive. The National Institutes of Health (NIH) has rejected this project once, but Cedars hasn't given up.

If You Are 30 or Older and Want Children

First, I am so glad that you have this book, because it means that you have a much better chance to experience the great joy parenthood brings. All of the information you'll read will help you decide what your first step will be. However, if you truly want to have a child, or children, whether you are single or not, you should at least take an FSH test, especially if you are 35 or over. If the results are at all borderline (10 to 15), see an expert, preferably a board certified reproductive endocrinologist, and while you are waiting for your appointment, turn to Chapter 5 for a review of what to expect and Chapter 4 to learn how to boost your chances for success. If your results are normal (under 10), read on, and make sure you take the appropriate steps in Chapter 4 to optimize your fertility potential for the future.

OLD BEFORE YOUR TIME

2.

Age is no barrier. It's a limitation you put on your mind.

—Jackie Joyner-Kersee

It is not how old you are, but how you are old.

—Marie Dressler

Young at Heart

Women are younger than they've ever been. Of course, some are more physically fit than others. Take Sister Madonna Buder, who started running at age 48 and competed in her first marathon at age 52—it was the grueling, uphill, Boston Marathon. That same year she decided to try a triathlon. Why stop at a 26.2-mile run? Why not add a 2.4-mile swim and a 112-mile bike race? Once she completed her first Ironman Triathlon, she was hooked. Since then, she's competed in a total of 300 triathlons. Now, at age 74, she says she's finished 30 of the world's top Ironman Triathlons, including 14 in Kona, Hawaii.

What Every Woman Needs to Know About...Her Biological Clock

She's not alone in her abilities. Fenya Crown evidently doesn't know that at 90 years old she should be sitting in her rocking chair rather than rocking and rolling to the finish line of a half marathon. Over the past two decades, she has run full-fledged marathons in China, France, Italy, and Canada. In November 2003 she dropped out of the Dublin Marathon after running 15 miles because so many spectators kept stopping her to take a picture. But rather than call it quits, she flew halfway across the globe to run that half marathon in sunny San Diego—essentially the other half of the race she started in Dublin. This remarkable woman took up running marathons at the age of 70!

There are other examples as well. Carol Sing, a woman from California swam the 21.5 miles across the English Channel, the day before her 58th birthday. She is the oldest woman to accomplish the daring feat. And then there's Mount Everest. Nancy Norris, 60 years young, hopes to become the oldest American woman to reach the summit, even though 63-year-old Tamae Watanabe of Japan snagged the world record for the oldest woman ever to climb the 29,035 foot peak. Unimpressed? It is estimated that there are about 120 much *younger* unrecovered corpses on Mount Everest.

All these women have succeeded in major physical tests of endurance, some over and over again. Their bodies are equipped to run, swim, and bike for miles, as well as climb straight up the highest mountain in the world, but they are anything but capable of doing one thing: making a baby. Indeed, there are perhaps hundreds, if not thousands of women 40 and over who run marathons and compete in triathlons every year, and their numbers are on the rise. These are healthy, strong, capable women. Yet, for all their energy, enthusiasm, and physical discipline, their reproductive capacity may as well be 6 feet under.

To me, this is a major paradox. Though I am no marathoner, nor do I ever expect to be, I consider myself healthy, relatively physically fit, and far from incapable of doing lots of things, including bearing and raising a child. So in my mind, biology is backward. Isn't it an absolute absurdity that I had a baby at 40, and couldn't get pregnant and stay pregnant again at 41? Lots of people, women included, will say, "Well, that's just the way it is, it's 'biology.'" Well, that isn't good enough for me. I wanted to know *why*. Why is biology out of whack when it comes to reproduction, especially today when women are living longer, and doing things such as running marathons at 90, triathlons at 73, and scaling Mount Everest at 63? This chapter along with the next will strive to answer the burning question: What is the biological clock, and why does it bite the dust halfway through life? Here are the answers I found.

Myths, Misconceptions, Misinformation

Everyone knows they have a biological clock, but few women stop and *really* think about what it is. We know we are supposed to get pregnant, and we know that at a certain time in our lives we will stop having our periods and presumably that is when we won't be able to have children anymore. Right? Wrong. On average women lose their fertility a solid 10 years before they stop menstruating—that is, reach menopause. I became angry when I started asking questions like these and finally got "expert" answers. For many months, I had been listening to women older than me, most of them already grandmothers, who kept saying, "Take your time, don't worry, you just had a baby." The fact is, the clock never stops, not when you are pregnant, not when you're breastfeeding, not when you are singing a lullaby to your naturally and easily conceived newborn.

My own mother was one of these older, and I thought wiser, women. (Don't get me wrong; she is wise, but just not in this particular area.) She knew we were struggling with trying to have our second child. Yet every time the subject came up she'd say, "Don't worry, so long as you have your period, you can get pregnant!" I finally asked her how she knew this, and she said her family doctor that delivered us (40-plus years ago!) told her so. I figured that source was a little shaky, but nobody else was telling me anything different.

Of course anyone who walks into an infertility clinic will quickly learn that you can have fabulously regular periods and be infertile, even if you've already had children. If your problem stems from an age-related fertility decline, you can continue to have predictable periods for years before they start becoming irregular due to the impending menopause. So, a period can't say whether you are fertile. In fact, it doesn't even mean you are ovulating, it simply means you are menstruating.

Many women also believe that because they are fit and feel young, they are fertile. Just about every reproductive endocrinologist I asked said their patients simply think they *should* be fertile because they take such good care of themselves. A healthy lifestyle may help you keep your clock running as long as it possibly can, but it does little or nothing to increase the amount of time you have to begin with. So if you don't smoke, avoid exposure to environmental toxins, and eat a healthy diet, your clock will run longer than it otherwise would, but so far, science indicates that all these great habits won't change the amount of time you innately have for reproduction. That's not to say living a healthy lifestyle makes no difference, on the contrary, this is, in fact, the only way to get the most out of your clock. Chapter 4 deals with all of this in-depth, and includes a way to best calculate the duration of your individual clock.

The Reproductive Reality

The American Infertility Association (AIA) has been actively trying to set the record straight for younger women. It is hardly an easy task. The AIA conducted a survey and found that only *one* woman out of more than 12,382 was able to correctly answer simple questions about the reproductive life cycle. Sadly, nearly 90 percent of the women overestimated by five to 10 years the age when fertility takes a steep irreversible nosedive. This miscalculation has had a disastrous impact on college-educated professional women who think they have most of their 30s and well into their 40s to have a family. The fact is, on average, a woman's fertility peaks from the late teens to the late 20s, then begins a gradual decline. Any day past 30 and you are dealing with a less than optimal biological clock. Initially the decline is hardly noticeable, but as more time passes, the steeper it gets.

Think of this downturn as a hillside. You start off walking relatively slowly and comfortably; it's a little faster than your normal gait, but you're steady down the hill. This trend continues until about age 35, when the slope begins to drop, forcing you to jog, then run. Sometime between age 40 and 42, the slope becomes more like a cliff. At this point, you are going to need a lot of gear, as well as perhaps some expert rock climbers to help you get where you want to go. And rock climbing might be easier with the best gear and assistance than trying to have a baby with the most high-tech treatment protocols and the best reproductive endocrinologists *after* you've hit this dramatic drop in fertility.

Of course there are exceptions to every rule, so some women may veer from these averages in either direction. The normal range for menopause is from the mid-40s to the late 50s, and this drastic fertility decline can begin from 10 to 12 years beforehand. Hence, many women still within the normal range can all of a sudden find themselves looking over this cliff and facing a next to impossible fertility battle anywhere from the mid-30s to the late 40s. Those women who delay childbearing until their 30s or early 40s, especially those on the earlier fringes, are most at risk for difficulties. Those fortunate enough to be blessed with a clock that runs fairly well into the 40s with a sharp decline after 45, and happen to still be working on their families, are those extremely rare later-in-life pregnancies that we hear about from time to time. However, it's important to realize that the vast majority of women fall somewhere in the middle of these ranges. Just for reference purposes, the average age of menopause is 51 and the average age of the severe decline in fertility (the cliff) is 41.

It's All About Your Ovaries: Egg Quantity and Egg Quality

From time to time I heard my biological clock ticking; it became loud and clear as I passed 35 and looked at 40 and found myself still single. However, I never knew that sound was coming from my ovaries. Now don't bend over and try to listen! Just know that what is happening in your ovaries will determine how long your clock ticks and how long you will be able to reproduce. First we'll look at what is understood about the biological clock in humans, and later we'll take a peek at new research in mice that may soon change our understanding of *how* the clock ticks.

The Quantity Issue

This next concept is so simple, yet few women are familiar with it. It is conventional wisdom and classical dogma (though the recent research just mentioned may change the concept) to all who deal with female reproduction, be they clinicians or researchers. The basic idea: you have all the eggs you will ever have at about 20 weeks gestation— while you are still growing in your mother's womb. At that point and throughout the rest of your life, you constantly *lose eggs* (that is, until you reach menopause, when you have essentially run out of them).

During fetal life, for reasons that are still unknown, you lose *most* of your eggs. David Keefe, M.D., director of two infertility clinics in New England and associate professor of obstetrics and gynecology at Brown University's Division of Biology and Medicine, makes this perfectly clear, "There is a massive die-off right at birth."

There are two theories as to why this happens. The current thinking is that during the birth process, the mother's hormones are at very high levels, and then all of a sudden they are withdrawn from the baby right at the same time the placenta is also removed. Keefe says, "There may be some effect from removing these two sources of hormones on the egg number, and once these hormones are gone, the baby loses 4 to 6 million eggs." The other theory is that there's something qualitatively different about these eggs and this is a kind of preprogrammed process that is internal. "It's like a checkpoint, a quality control step, where those eggs that are of lesser quality just die at birth rather than being carried throughout life. It's all poorly understood. What we do know is the eggs die," adds Keefe.

Here are the numbers according to the dogma. A female fetus has 6 to 7 million eggs at 20 weeks development. When born, that number drops to just 1 to 2 million, and by the time a girl gets her first period, she is left with about 300,000 viable eggs from which to produce offspring. A woman's fertility, it appears, begins declining almost as soon as she is formed. However, the 300,000 eggs a girl has to start her reproductive years are what matter most. It would seem, even with this vast number of eggs, that women should have no problem reproducing well into middle age and beyond. But the problem is twofold. Each month, you lose many eggs, and at a certain age, this decline in egg *quantity* seems to correspond with a drop in egg *quality*.

Keefe says to think of eggs as little bubbles that spring up constantly from a storage depot inside the ovary. On most days, because there's no hormone available or there's some inherent defect in them, just like bubbles, they disappear. On the days when hormone is circulating in your system—that is, the menstrual cycle has begun—then one or occasionally two eggs are rescued from certain death, and they rise out of the group, mature, and finally become the ovulated eggs. These eggs are lost too if they are never fertilized. But the important point is all of your ovulated eggs amount to next to nothing in the big picture. According to Keefe, "You lose eggs every day. The menstrual cycle is just imposed on this chronic, tonic, persistent, incessant loss. It's totally depressing when you think about it, but that's the reality of it."

The Quality Issue

Here's a little known, but I think pretty astounding, bit of research to get you thinking about the quantity/quality issue and how it may interact with age. A University of California, Davis, longevity researcher transplanted much younger ovaries into older mice. Drum roll please.... The older mice lived 40 percent longer than the normal control group! These 11-month old females, which would be equivalent to 50-year-old women, also started their menstrual cycles again, and continued their reproductive cycles several months beyond the age they would normally stop reproducing. Though the study was done in mice, it demonstrates that younger mammalian ovaries are likely better ovaries, even if they aren't yours to begin with!

Eggs in Waiting

Getting back to *your* eggs...remember, according to the textbooks, they've all been there since before you were born, and each one of them also began to prepare for ovulation back in your mother's womb. (Again, the new research discussed at the end of this chapter could alter this.) However, they also all stopped the process before you were born. So all the eggs you started your reproductive years with remained in a kind of state of suspended animation for many years, and those you currently have are still in this state. One or two of the group that bubble up from that reservoir each month will go on to ovulation, and perhaps fertilization. Basically, the immature egg selected for ovulation goes through a maturation process necessary for it to unite with a sperm cell.

However, to understand fully why older eggs don't work as well as younger eggs, you have to realize that this maturation process is not easy. Imagine the egg and all its inner parts performing an incredibly delicate yet strenuous choreography akin to a stage full of ballet dancers executing precision moves in unison, perfectly timed to reach the

What Every Woman Needs to Know About...Her Biological Clock

finale flawlessly—no bumping, tripping, or ending up where you're not supposed to be. And this group of dancers must perform this exact ballet, not once but twice before the show is over. Now imagine that rather than 20-year-old ballet dancers, they are all pushing 40 or older—you get the picture!

This delicate dance is called *meiosis*. It is a very tricky process within the egg, and it has to be performed whenever the egg is called upon to do so. That means your egg might be 25, 33, or 42 years old when it's time to swing into action. It's no great leap to imagine, that a 35- or 40-year-old egg may have a little more trouble completing the task than an a younger egg. However, a single misstep can mean the demise of the egg or if it gets that far, the embryo, or even the fetus.

Here's how the process works. We all have 46 pairs of chromosomes in our cells, one set from mom, one from dad. However, an egg has to have half that number (23) so it can unite with a sperm, which also has half, to bring the combined number back to the normal 46. When an egg is selected for ovulation, however, it has *four* times the number of chromosomes it needs to unite with a sperm. Back in fetal life the chromosomes actually replicated, then froze in that state of suspended animation. In order for the egg to reduce this number, it has to go through two separate divisions and discard a total of three sets of chromosomes. During each division, it must form a structure to coordinate all the action, plus a critical scaffolding for the chromosomes to line up on and separate along. This scaffolding is called the spindle.

In the first division, tiny filament-like structures form in the spindle so that two sets of 46 chromosomes can arrange themselves side by side, then split up and separate. (You've no doubt seen something like this if you've ever been to a ballet—the Radio City Rockettes come to mind too!) One set of chromosomes stays in what will eventually become the ovulated egg, and the other set is sent out of the egg in a much smaller structure called a first polar body. The second division is comprised of two portions and only begins if a sperm cell penetrates the egg to begin fertilization. The first polar body divides again; two smaller polar bodies each with 23 pairs of chromosomes are just discarded. However, what happens in the larger cell is crucial to successful fertilization. At this time another spindle is formed and the 46 chromosomes again line up on it, then split into 23 pairs

46

and start separating from each other along the spindle filaments, also known as microtubules. This portion is analogous to the second performance.

These 23 pairs of chromosomes are exact copies of each other. They carry the genes, which determine everything from hair color to height to musical ability. Once the separation is complete, another small polar body is discarded but the much larger and very mature egg retains the other 23 pairs, which will be the mother's contribution to the embryo as fertilization continues. The complementary 23 pairs will come from the father's side—the sperm. So the egg essentially discarded three sets of chromosomes without missing a beat, then during fertilization, it has to find and organize all the sperm's duplicate chromosomes and match them exactly with each of the egg's—in perfect unison. I'm exhausted just writing about it! Hopefully you now realize that older, or less than perfectly fit, eggs simply don't perform all these precision moves as well as eggs that are either younger or in tip-top shape.

Spinster Spindles

Now that you have the basics, here is what some of the most current science has revealed about what may be going wrong in older eggs. The spindle plays a major role because it is crucial to the proper separation of the chromosomes during both stages of meiosis. Many studies have shown that the eggs of older women either don't have spindles, they are malformed, or they just don't work very well. Sometimes spindles appear normal, but on closer examination, the chromosomes aren't able to do their dance. They may not separate or move properly along the spindle, or a chromosome gets left behind or gets stuck, leaving an extra one in the final mature egg. The scientific word for these klutzy dance steps is "nondisjunction," and the technical word that describes the mistake that results is "aneuploidy."

Exactly what causes nondisjunction, whether it is faulty scaffolding or a mishap in the mechanisms that coordinate the action, remains to be determined. It appears the cause may be a combination of both structure and function gone awry. One study showed the spindles in 79 percent of the eggs from older women ages 40 to 45 had abnormal microtubules (filaments that the chromosomes travel along) and one or more misplaced chromosomes. Only 17 percent of the eggs from the younger group ages 20 to 25 had any of these defects.

Other studies have looked at living, maturing eggs undergoing in vitro fertilization. Using a special microscope, called a Polscope, that is able to look *inside* a living egg, two groups of researchers have shown more visible, sturdy spindles mean better embryos. One of these studies found quality embryos in 64 percent of eggs with visible spindles, and quality embryos in only 36 percent of eggs without visible spindles. Another study showed that 53 percent of eggs with spindles developed for six straight days in vitro, whereas only 29 percent without spindles made it that far. These researchers concluded that the presence of a well-structured spindle amounts to better function, and therefore more viable embryos.

Doomed From the Start?

Some experts believe that older eggs may be at a disadvantage from the day they were formed. These researchers adhere to what's called the "production line theory." The theory goes like this. Back when you were just a bunch of cells beginning to differentiate into real organs, about five to 10 so-called "germ cells" came along and created your eggs. As these eggs are being created, they are formed in a kind of production line. The eggs formed first, duplicate themselves and become more eggs, then they replicate again and become more eggs, and so on. This production line theory postulates that the eggs that are ovulated first, that is, earlier in reproductive life, are those that came off this production line first. The key to understanding this theory is that these first or *earlier* ovulated eggs went through *fewer* duplications. They are copies of copies, rather than copies of copies of copies, etc. The latter are those you would ovulate later in life, and they would therefore be a little more worn out. Think of what happens when you make too many copies of a videotape—the picture isn't as crisp, and the more copies, the worse the picture.

This theory holds that the eggs that bubble up when your biological clock is brand new and working like a charm are chosen because they are higher quality; and those that bubble up later in life are the leftovers, the bottom of the barrel, so to speak.

However, there are other schools of thought as well. Another theory suggests the bubbling up and subsequent selection of the ovulated egg during the cycle has to do with genetics and some sort of signaling mechanism and has nothing to do with when the eggs were formed during fetal life. However, neither of these theories may be correct, or will at least have to be modified, if very recent research on mouse egg production holds true for humans. More on this in a moment.

Another bit of information that uncovers further evidence that old eggs may be doomed from the start relates to how the genes from your mother and father are combined within your egg cells. During egg production, when duplicate pairs of chromosomes from your mother and father come together before they divide into two separate cells, they perform a rather important and somewhat sensual dance. These chromosomes wrap around each other at the same place, and pieces literally snap apart and fuse at the same place on the other chromosome. For example, the chromosome carrying a short stature gene from your mother's side will fuse onto the chromosome pair from your father's side—and his tall stature gene will take the empty place on the chromosome from your mother's side. The same genes basically switch sides. This "crossing over" is called a chiasma.

The result is that the traits that happen to be on the 23 pairs of chromosomes contained in the ovulated egg is anyone's guess. Early in fetal life, all the genes you have from your mother and father literally get shuffled within your eggs as they are being created. This is why when you have children, each one is different— possibly one short, one tall. They do not carry the same exact set of chromosomes that you or your husband have; each child is a unique combination of the genes from both sides of your families. This is what makes each person a true individual, unlike any other.

Okay, this is all very interesting, but how does it relate to aging eggs? It turns out that babies that are born with chromosomal disorders that result from mistakes of meiosis, or nondisjunction, such as Down syndrome, have fewer of these genetic crossovers, or chiasmata, in their chromosomes; they have less genetic variability. It appears then that eggs that are ovulated later, which definitely have a higher risk of chromosomal abnormalities, also have less gene shuffling. Why this occurs is unclear. It may be that those eggs last off the production line have less ability to perform this gene shuffling, or some mechanism inhibits this process as the eggs are forming, resulting in less than perfect eggs, which are simply not selected until later in life. Still, it appears that the older you are, the less genetic

49

variability your eggs have, and the better the chances they will not produce a baby.

Damage Over Time

There are a number of other insults that, over time, damage your eggs. A master of analogies, David Keefe says, "It's just like your pocketbook. It doesn't look the same 15 years after you bought it—stuff happens to it, it gets worn down." Of course, we generally don't keep pocketbooks for 15 years, but given how they look after a few months we can just imagine! So, even though eggs are somewhat protected inside the ovaries, given they sit there for so long, they do get a bit worn.

How does this happen? Things that cause all of the cells in our bodies to age also impact eggs. For instance, the constant bombardment of gamma radiation from the sun and stars knocks out DNA. Cells can repair this DNA damage, but over time the wear and tear accumulates and is permanent. This destruction happens inside the egg's nucleus, where all of our chromosomes are located, where there is some ability to repair the damage, and it also takes place in the fluid and structures containing DNA surrounding the nucleus, where there isn't much damage control going on. Keefe's lab has proposed that these tiny structures called mitochondria, which contain their own separate DNA, accumulate damage.

The mitochondria—known as the powerhouses of the cell—give the egg the energy to do all it needs to do. However, mitochondrial DNA is very susceptible to damage because these compact structures lack a good repair mechanism. "These tiny power plants are very dense in terms of the amount of information they have. They have very little wasted DNA; just about every part of the DNA encodes important information. So damage may be very detrimental to the egg cell," says Keefe who has seen mutations in the mitochondrial DNA in eggs from older women.

Others argue that the overall damage resulting from *oxidation* is far more insidious to aging eggs. Reactive oxygen molecules, which are highly unstable, are popularly known as "free radicals." These molecules are natural by-products of metabolism within the body. Just like your furnace, your body cells burn food as fuel to keep you going, and in the process, these free radicals are created. All cells that are alive, including egg cells, will naturally accumulate damage due to free radicals in DNA, whether in the nucleus or mitochondria, as well as in proteins and fats inside cells.

But there are other environmental causes of oxidative damage in egg cells. One major source that has been documented many times is tobacco smoke. Smoking will damage and kill so many eggs that it will cause an earlier menopause. Secondhand smoke may have an effect as well, though not as severe. Also, some studies have suggested that the eggs in a female fetus, whose mother smokes, may be subject to this kind of damage as well. Researchers theorize that these baby girls may start life with fewer eggs and may run out sooner, leading to "unexplained" infertility, and possibly an earlier menopause. Other environmental sources of oxidative damage that can chip away at your eggs and slowly rust your clock, include workplace toxins, natural arsenic as well as arsenic-treated wood, pesticides, various solvents, PCBs, and even household hazardous materials. See Chapter 4 for a comprehensive look at smoking and other environmental hazards, and the damage they can cause.

The Long and Short of Telomeres

Telomeres are repetitive sequences of DNA that cap and protect the ends of chromosomes. It has been known for some time that when cells divide, causing chromosomes to duplicate, telomeres get shorter. The more a cell divides, then, the shorter the telomeres become. Once they are reduced to a certain point, the cells can no longer divide, and they die. In animal models, research has shown that well-functioning telomeres on the chromosomes inside eggs, result in good spindle formation and proper separation of chromosomes, leading to viable mature eggs and embryos.

Keefe believes telomeres hold the key to why all the quality issues previously mentioned produce older eggs that are so prone to defects, and therefore infertility problems and miscarriages. Keefe first studied telomeres in mice and found that when researchers purposely shortened telomeres in the eggs of mice, many of the eggs died, and those that survived created abnormal spindles. The embryos subsequently created from these eggs also developed abnormally. Because the eggs and embryos in these experimental mice looked remarkably like those of older women undergoing in vitro fertilization, Keefe decided to look at the telomeres inside human eggs.

His team focused on spare human eggs donated by patients. It was a small study, but nevertheless, the findings proved unmistakable. They examined 43 eggs that were retrieved but not fertilized. They used a technique that paints the telomeres with a light-emitting molecule, which can be measured by a detector on a microscope. They found the telomeres were shortest in the eggs from women who failed IVF, compared to those who succeeded and got pregnant. In fact, there wasn't a single pregnancy when the telomeres dipped below a certain length. All of the normal predictors of infertility, even age, were similar among these patients; the overriding difference among their eggs was telomere length.

Keefe believes shortened telomeres explain why later in life women's eggs are basically *old.* If the production line theory is true, it makes sense that the last eggs to exit and be used would have shorter telomeres. The reason is simple: they have been through the most cell divisions—remember the copies of copies of copies of copies? Each time the eggs divided, they lost a little bit of telomere length; those that were created at the back end of the production line would then have shorter telomeres to begin with.

Other research has shown that telomeres are important for the lining up of the chromosomes to form chiasma. Keefe's team recently demonstrated that purposely shortening telomeres in mice cuts the number of chiasma in half. So basically, if many divisions mean shorter telomeres, then it may also mean fewer chiasma; neither is good for eggs. According to Keefe, "This is the so-called 'first hit' that certain eggs will be subject to, and we think these are the ones that are ovulated later in life."

However, combine that with the "second hit" that these eggs encounter just by hanging around in the body so long, and you have a recipe for plummeting egg quality as we age. The second hit is really all the oxidative damage that egg cells are subjected to due to natural metabolism; outside forces, such as natural radiation; plus the other damaging agents we can control, such as tobacco smoke, or arsenic exposure, and those we often can't control such as PCBs or pesticides. "It appears that older eggs are subject to a 'double whammy'; first in fetal life and then over time as women age. I believe a woman's fertility will be shown to be as good as the shortest telomere from a single egg," adds Keefe.

Other Undeniable Evidence

The Incredible Shrinking Ovary

Perhaps the most obvious evidence that quantity of eggs decreases as we age is that the organ that holds them *shrinks*. I know this is not a very pleasant thought, and the first time I read it, I cringed. But the fact is, one of the tests for reproductive aging is "ovarian volume." The less volume, the fewer eggs inside. Young ovaries are plump because they are chock full of eggs, but over time, they begin to deflate. This is something a good reproductive endocrinologist can detect using a vaginal ultrasound. A family doctor may not be able to notice a difference until much later.

Pre-implantation Genetic Diagnosis (PGD)

This new technology has helped countless couples have healthy, normal babies. It has also helped many others halt emotionally difficult and financially draining treatment because they learned that continuing would be essentially futile. Pre-implantation genetic diagnosis, or PGD, can screen growing cells for genetic defects very early in embryonic life. It involves taking a single cell from a recently fertilized embryo and peering inside it at its chromosomes. It does pretty much the same thing that an amniocentesis does—only five months sooner. The advantage with PGD is you don't have to wait until you are nearly halfway through a pregnancy to learn that the baby may have a devastating genetic disease; in fact, you never have to become pregnant with a baby that has a major genetic problem. As you can imagine, this is a wonderful advance for people who are at greater risk of passing along an inherited disease, or women of advanced age who want to know their embryos are healthy before they are transferred to their wombs.

This technique, however, also provides undeniable evidence that older eggs have a much higher incidence of chromosomal problems. One set of studies examined just six out of the 23 chromosomes, and found that up to 70 percent of the older eggs had signs of nondisjunction, that is, either a missing or an extra chromosome. PGD has shown the older a woman is, the more aneuploidy (chromosome defects) present. Depending on the severity, some defects may be hardly noticeable; fertilization fails and an embryo doesn't even develop; or a woman has a miscarriage and doesn't know it—she'll simply get a period either on time or a few days late. Other chromosomal errors, however, can lead to later, very apparent miscarriages, a baby born with Down syndrome, or another genetic disorder.

Everyone knows the probability of Down syndrome rises with age. This is direct evidence of aneuploidy at work. In Down syndrome, also called Trisomy 21, there is an extra chromosome 21—for some reason it gets stuck and is never expelled from the cell that becomes the egg. Therefore, when the sperm unites and brings in its complementary chromosome 21, there are three copies, rather than the normal two. Looking at the big picture, this is one of the less damaging mistakes, because it still results in a baby, but of course, for the parents, it can be heart wrenching. Miscarriage tissue from older women also shows high rates of aneuploidy; one clinic director reported that well over 90 percent of miscarriages he's seen in older women involve chromosomal problems.

Donor Eggs Work

Just 20 years ago, nobody really knew whether the slowing of the biological clock was a function of the uterus, the endocrine system, or the ovaries. It wasn't until a handful of clinics began trying to help their infertile patients with the use of donated eggs that it became clear it was indeed the ovaries. One of the first donor egg programs started in 1988 at the Albert Einstein College of Medicine in New York City. Dr. Michael Feinman, now the director of the Huntington Reproductive Center in California, began the program in New York. "No one had really crossed the line yet, to seek volunteer egg donors, so it wasn't so much a race to see who would be first, it was where do we get eggs?" Feinman says it was a fortunate coincidence that just upstairs from his clinic was another where women could get their tubes tied. "We started approaching the tubal ligation patients to donate eggs while they were having their procedure. They were mostly women who had children, and who obviously didn't want more children. They were an ideal pool of patients. A relatively small number agreed, but it was enough to get us started, and keep our program going," says Feinman.

Around the same time, a clinic on the West Coast also began pushing the frontiers of egg donation. Dr. Richard Paulson has remained at the forefront of this increasingly popular service, and admits, "We had no idea that egg donation was going to help women that are getting older. It was a serendipitous finding."

At the time, doctors were using donor eggs to treat women with premature ovarian failure; these are women whose fertility drops irreversibly before age 40. Egg donation was originally designed for them. In fact, in Paulson's clinic, all of the women had to be *under* 40 years old in order to be considered for the upstart egg donation program. However, some had to wait so long for egg donors, they turned 40 in the meantime. Paulson and his team decided to allow them to continue, and then began treating others who turned 41 and 42. Eventually what was happening sunk in, says Paulson, "There was an 'aha' moment—they were getting pregnant at the same rate as the younger women!"

That observation opened the floodgates. Today, it is fairly commonplace for women in their 40s and even early 50s to have babies through egg donation. The reason is simple: it works! Furthermore, it isn't exactly clear when a woman's body becomes *unable* to carry a baby. There have been a few births to women in their *60s*. These births demonstrate two things: your eggs determine your biological clock, they drive the system, they do the ticking; and given good *young* eggs, your body and your reproductive system will remain able to create life well past menopause.

New Discovery Tinkers With Biological Clock

For decades researchers and physicians alike based their belief that a woman has all the eggs she'll ever have at birth on scientific data that appeared correct—but may not be. A new study could completely revise that belief. Though the research was done in mice, it may eventually alter much of what you just read. If it does, however, it's important to note it will have essentially no impact on the ultimate outcome and time frame for the biological clock. Still, according to lead author of the study, Jonathan Tilly, Ph.D., of the Vincent Center for Reproductive Biology at Massachusetts General Hospital (MGH), "It makes you rethink *how* the clock ticks."

Tilly and his team set out to get a better handle on the numbers of eggs lost during development and adulthood in mice, because this had never been precisely calculated before. What they came up with didn't make sense. They discovered that tremendous amounts of eggs were dying and being cleared away from mouse ovaries in short order. In fact, so many eggs were disappearing (a process called *atresia*) that researchers estimated the ovaries should have failed completely within just two weeks—but they didn't. In fact, the number of eggs remained static. They kept counting to make sure they were correct, and finally had no choice but to consider the notion that *new* eggs were being manufactured to replace those being lost. This idea completely contradicts the classical belief that mice and other mammals possess a fixed number of eggs at birth and are incapable of generating new ones in adulthood. "Once we did the clearance experiments and we measured how quickly these things [eggs] get flushed out, that's when we knew we really had the dogma by the tail—it was wrong!" exclaims Tilly.

Impact on Our Understanding of the Clock

Several additional experiments appear to confirm that *new* eggs are being generated in the mouse ovary. Researchers showed that both mitosis and meiosis are occurring in *adult* ovaries indicating *stem cells* are likely at work producing the new eggs; both processes were thought to have only occurred in fetal life during ovary development. The MGH team has also happened upon a unique strain of mouse that developed 20 percent more eggs in adulthood than they had at birth! Tilly adds, "It all made sense to us because the numbers don't lie, numbers are numbers." He says there's every reason to believe the same mechanism is at work in primates, including humans.

Recently, Tilly's team announced further advances at a scientific conference in Europe. According to reports, they have isolated up to 200 of these egg-producing cells from a single mouse ovary, and have shown that these cells contain genetic markers that indicate they are indeed stem cells capable of creating mouse eggs. In addition, the team revealed they may have discovered a gene that regulates the stem cells. When they knocked out this gene, the resulting mice had 40 percent more eggs in their ovaries than normal. Finally, they have developed a molecule that somehow forces the stem cells to produce more eggs; when they injected it into female mice just before puberty, they produced nearly double the normal number of follicles.

This means much of the science on the biological clock and how it works will likely be revisited, including Tilly's own previous research. If it turns out new eggs are being made in women, and it is not the actual age of the *eggs* that results in poor quality, what it could mean is that the age of the *stem cells*, and their capacity to manufacture healthy eggs wanes as the clock slows. So, even if we are making new eggs, these eggs are not as high quality as they once were because the production pipeline—that is, the stem cells—could be dying off, and/or becoming much less efficient with time. Tilly explains, "Obviously, if they are pushing eggs into the human ovary from birth to the age of 50, they've been dividing quite a lot—and we don't think there are a lot of these stem cells to begin with. So maybe they're failing to perform their function, and that's seen clinically two ways, one there are fewer eggs coming out, and the eggs that are coming out are poorer quality."

In fact, Tilly agrees that the idea of active ovarian stem cells might further explain the production line theory, as well as the how additional internal and external insults wreak havoc on eggs, and therefore the biological clock. These processes, including the continued replication (copies of copies of copies) and radiation and free radical insults (natural, as well as environmental exposures), rather than acting on the individual *eggs* that were thought to remain in the ovary over a woman's reproductive lifespan, may instead be doing their damage to the individual *stem cells* producing the eggs. Further research is necessary to explore these possibilities, but if proven to be true, the biological clock may wind down because of aging stem cells that are dying off and/or producing poor quality eggs, rather than due to aging eggs.

If this is the case, and stem cells are confirmed in human ovaries, and they can be manipulated as they have been recently in mice, they could then be targeted for new potentially breakthrough treatment possibilities. According to Tilly, "If the ovaries can be revived or restored even for a few years, obviously you can begin to think about not only extending fertility in women, but also potentially even delaying the menopause." (See Chapter 7 for more on the exciting research that may come out of this finding.)

Backward Biology

3.

> *I am so angry.*
> *I'm in great shape, I run every day, I've finally found the right man,*
> *and we're so much in love, but thanks to this ridiculous clock, I've run*
> *out of time to have children.*
>
> —Jane, age 45

> *Screw biology!*
> *I want a child, and I'll do anything I can to make that possible. Mother*
> *Nature should be ashamed of herself; she's got a lot of nerve telling*
> *me I can't have a family because I arrived a little too late!*
>
> —Vicki, age 38

> *Evolution has got it wrong these days. The species is losing out on lots*
> *of highly effective, bright people that will never be born—it's not like*
> *we all have six or 10 kids already. We just want one.*
>
> —Bob, husband of Morgan, 40

Millennium Women With a Stone Age Clock

Did I mention to you that I think the biological clock is out of whack? Okay, maybe women who have had four kids before age 25 wouldn't agree, but chances are, if you are reading this, you likely think so too. I got my first period at age 11—does that make sense today? Absolutely not! Anybody who tells you otherwise either never had a daughter or never will have one. Granted, the first couple of years of menstruation are generally infertile, however, that would have put me at say 13 or 14, when I could have started having children. At the time, I was way too busy finishing middle school, or deciding whether I should join the track team or cheerleading squad my first year in high school. However, according to Mother Nature, that's when I should have started reproducing.

Fast-forward to college and the career beyond. Most women end up spending a lot of their lives preventing pregnancy; in my case that was certainly true, and just when I was ready to finally complete my family, WHAM! Not a chance. The clock has stopped, Cara—too bad, you can blame it on *biology*. Well, if we blamed cancer on biology we wouldn't be curing anybody. If we blamed heart disease on biology, there wouldn't be pacemakers, defibrillators, or heart transplants. If we blamed bad eyesight on biology, we'd all be squinting and bumping into each other. The point is that we are completely and totally all about *biology*, but we can change it, and we can make it better. I feel the same about this wacky, antiquated, inflexible clock. If it's broken, let's fix it. And I don't mean give women a list of egg donor agencies; I mean *really* fix it.

We've conquered contraception with a pill, we've even conquered erectile dysfunction in 80-year-old men, can we not figure out a way to suspend our fertility until we want to use it? At the very least, isn't there a way to reenergize slightly older eggs so we can pass on our genes at age 40 or 45? Surely, evolution would prefer that to no genetic legacy at all.

Unfortunately, at the moment, evolution could care less about whether we beat our clocks or remain childless. Like the clock itself, evolution marches to the beat of its own drummer. We are a product of a score this drummer decided upon 1 or 2 million years ago. As you

60

will see in the rest of this chapter, there remains quite a division among anthropologists, evolutionary biologists, and other experts as to what exactly this drummer drummed up. That is, there are two basic schools of thought relative to why we evolved a reproductive system that stops when we are generally speaking, still so young and full of life. These two camps agree on little but the fact that an abrupt human reproductive decline leading to menopause in midlife is a mystery worth exploring.

No comprehensive look at the biological clock would be complete without a glance at where this clock may have come from, and why. Though facing a slowing clock is a trauma best avoided, either theory, along with their spin-offs presented here, provides a reasonable foundation for understanding why such an unforgiving deadline exists.

The Antiquated Clock

Scientists agree our biological clock is the same now as it's been since we were hit over the head and dragged into caves to start our families. The evolutionary pressures that molded our clocks may have begun as far back as our earliest ancestors first roamed the Earth—4 to 5 million years ago. If it took at least a few million years of evolution for our clock to take its present form, you can bet it won't be changing on its own any time soon. Evolution is a painstakingly slow process.

However, what has changed is the way we live, and even more importantly, how long we live. Gone are the prehistoric predators that would just as soon dine on a human as an antelope; gone are the mud or grass huts that severe weather would pulverize; gone are many fatal infectious diseases that would wipe out entire populations. Today, we can avoid many external causes of death that would constantly knock on the doors of our bipedal ancestors, as well as even our grandparents, great-grandparents, and their parents. Not only have these causes of death vanished, but we now know how to avoid many of the contemporary causes of death: we can stop smoking to avoid lung disease; we can eat a better diet to prevent heart disease; we can have regular cancer screenings to catch a tumor and treat it before it's too late; we can strap on our seatbelts. The list goes on.

According to the Centers for Disease Control (CDC), the 10 greatest public health achievements in the 20th century include vaccination, motor-vehicle safety, control of infectious diseases, and recognition of tobacco use as a health hazard. All of these improvements have lead to longer, healthier lives among Americans. Indeed, Americans born today can expect to live at least 30 years longer than in 1900. The CDC attributes about 25 years of this gain to advances in public health.

Back in 1900, a baby girl could anticipate living to age 48, but by 1950, the average life expectancy jumped to 71. Since then, there has been a steady increase of about one to two years per decade: in 1990 she could expect to live to 78.8; and in 2001, life expectancy for a newborn girl jumped to 79.8 years. Just for the record, the life expectancy for American males has also increased steadily, though as of 2001, it still lags about five years behind women, at 74.4. Interestingly, if a woman was already 75 in 2001, on average she could expect to make it to 87—another 12 years!

This is hardly an American phenomenon. Life expectancies have increased, and are expected to continue to increase throughout the world. In France, over the past 50 years (from 1950 to 1998), life expectancy increased 13 years to nearly 83 years old for women; among women in Sweden, average life expectancy increased almost 10 years to 82; and in Egypt there was more than a 20-year jump, from 43.6 to 64.1 years over the same time period. However, the gold medal for life expectancy goes to Japan, which also increased 20 years to 83.3 years for women.

Data has shown that in Japan's state of Okinawa, people live the longest in the world. Researchers at Harvard Medical School and Okinawa International University surveyed the entire population of this chain of 44 inhabited islands alongside the Japan main island, and identified 427 people who have reached at least 100 years of age. This represents a prevalence of 33.6 centenarians per 100,000 people—the highest concentration of centenarians in the world, documented with a reliable database. And guess what? More than 85 percent are women!

Let's think about this. If the average age of menopause remains nearly constant, and if these life expectancies continue upward, many women will be spending nearly 40 years of life unable to reproduce. So far, my own mother has spent 37 years *not* reproducing. If we believe what Darwin taught us (most agree he was right about most things evolution), that the survival of our species is all about passing as many of our genes as possible to the next generation, then how can living 30, 40, possibly even 50 years without any ability to reproduce be a good strategy?

One evolutionary theory of this early reproductive senescence (decline in fertility leading to menopause) says it is a perfectly appropriate strategy to ensure your genetic code is handed over to future generations, the other says that's bunk. There is very little middle ground among the proponents of each theory. Nevertheless, both explanations are intriguing. I will present them with as little bias as possible, as I have yet to completely decide which camp makes the most sense. Science isn't perfect, and this is a field of study still in its infancy...no pun intended!

Is the Slowing Clock an Adaptation?

When evolutionary biologists are looking for answers, they often search for a good reason why a trait exists. For example, why do cats have claws? Obviously, during the cat's evolution, those individuals in a population that grew the sharpest claws caught the most food, were better able to defend themselves, and were possibly better at climbing trees to escape their enemies. So cats with sharp claws lived, and could reproduce kittens with sharp claws, and they lived, and could reproduce more sharp-clawed kittens, and so on. This is the basic idea behind the process of "natural selection," which leads to adaptations. Hence, cats have adapted sharp claws. Many scientists believe the same kind of mechanism led to a biological clock that starts slowing in the first quarter of life, and then completely stops with decades of life still to go.

Reproductive Altruism

Those who adhere to this view believe reproductive senescence and menopause have a purpose. They believe when our prehistoric foremothers relinquished reproduction early, it helped future generations survive. During these evolutionary times, when there was no means of contraception, women bore many children. Few of them lived, of course; however, all children had a better chance to make it to adulthood if their mothers' also remained alive.

If ancient mothers were subjected to giving birth later and later in life, this camp believes, they risked dying due to the difficulties of childbirth. These mothers would have left young orphans, who also likely would have died. Childbirth later in life, therefore, could be fatal to a woman. Women who had genes that allowed them to become pregnant at an advanced age often died, and so did her offspring. So very few of these children lived to pass along these "later reproduction" genes. To give you a visual, think about giving birth at an advanced age if you lived in a hut in the hills of France during the Dark Ages. There were no blood transfusions, no IVs, no medications; if there was a problem, chances are you would die. Not very pleasant, and it could cost your life. During ancient times, there was either horrendous, often dangerous, medical care, or none at all. Women of today face similar risks as they age, especially at significantly advanced ages, but they have the benefit of some of the best medical care the 21st century has to offer.

Now to understand the flip side of the adaptation theory, consider the mothers who *lost* their ability to reproduce early in life and never faced the age-related increased dangers of childbirth. They lived to raise the children they already had. These children, therefore, also survived to pass along these "age-related-infertility-is-a-good-thing," or "early menopause-is-a-good-thing" genes. So, halting reproduction when the risk of childbirth proved minimal was a trait that was intentionally "selected." Based on this theory, our early wind down to menopause may have emerged as a positive adaptation called *reproductive altruism*.

Basically, it means women gave up their own fertility to benefit the fertility of their offspring. The classic example occurs in ants and some other insects such as bees. The drones, or workers, sacrifice everything for the reproductive success of the queen. All they do is bring food to her, so there's no time for their own reproduction. They never reproduce; they spend their entire little lives making sure the queen is nourished, so she can do all the reproducing.

The idea in humans is that women sacrifice their own reproductive success early on, so they stick around to see that their children survive and reproduce. This way, a mother is better able take care of her genetic heritage in the offspring she already has, and make sure these family genes will continue to be passed into the future. In fact, some who adhere to this theory also believe that even if an older mother survived childbirth and had a baby, the energy she would have to expend to care for him or her meant her other offspring would suffer, perhaps to the point of malnutrition and death. In natural selection terms, that trade-off would not be worth it; better to invest in what you have than start caring for a totally dependent newborn. Of course, if this older mom with other kids eventually died before the newborn could survive on its own, she would have lost the other children, lost the newborn, and therefore spent nearly all of her life trying to pass on her genes and completely failed. Her late-in-life baby-making genes would be gone forever. Think about it, back in these dangerous times, if your ovaries shut down, and you stopped making fertile eggs at 30, you (and your genes) might be much better off than your lady friend who continued to be fertile, had more little ones, and then died from something such as childbirth, or a hungry bear.

This mechanism has also been reported in a number of highly social long-lived mammalian species, such as whales and dolphins; large land mammals, such as elephants; and primates. Also, more than a hundred species of monkeys and apes show evidence of reproductive altruism. In the journal *Fertility and Sterility*, Dr. David Keefe, a proponent of the reproductive altruism adaptation theory, writes: "They include the most biologically successful species that ever existed, indicating the important survival value conferred by reproductive altruism." He argues part of the reason this theory is advantageous to humans and other long-lived mammals is we produce relatively few offspring, compared to short-lived mammals such as rabbits or rodents, and we invest a tremendous amount of time in bringing them up. The fewer offspring, the longer a mother generally needs to make sure her children survive. If she stops reproducing, she has more time to spend with the children she already has.

The Grandmother Hypothesis, or "Go Grandma!"

The Grandmother Hypothesis (GMH) takes reproductive altruism one step further. This theory is aligned with the adaptation theory, but in addition, proposes that infertile older women—that is, grandmothers—had long lives after their reproductive years because they had a most important role to play. The GMH suggests *grandmothers* made a huge difference in making sure the family's genes made it to the next generation and beyond, and were instrumental in the evolution of our biological clock, and even our species.

What Every Woman Needs to Know About...Her Biological Clock

Is grandma responsible for making us human as opposed to ape-like? That's the latest twist on the GMH. University of Utah anthropologist Kristen Hawkes, Ph.D., who originally proposed the theory, says during our evolution, one thing separated us from our closest relatives, the great apes—our grandmothers! She writes in the *American Journal of Human Biology*, "A novel role for grandmothers underlies the shift from an ape-like ancestral pattern to one more like our own in the first widely successful members of genus Homo." Basically, Hawkes argues that these first non-reproducing grandmas were expert providers. Because they weren't caring for their own offspring anymore, they could help feed their daughters, and *their* children. That way, grandma's daughters could concentrate on newborn after newborn—thus passing on grandma's genes—including the quit-reproducing-early genes. Over eons, this pattern selected for a sudden decline in fertility, allowed women to concentrate on the children they already had, and eventually created long-lived infertile grandmothers who could feed the grandchildren while their daughters concentrated on having more babies.

Hawkes bases this theory on the Hadza people, a tribe of foragers in northern Tanzania. The government has tried to help these people become farmers, but they seem to prefer the bush, where there is plenty of fruits, honey, and tubers. It turns out that after careful study, it is the old women that ultimately keep everyone fed. In this primitive, though contemporary society, about one-third of women live beyond childbearing age, and they spend much of their time foraging for food. By the age of 5, children also gather their own food, primarily fruit that is easy for them to find and pick. However, during the dry spells, when fruit is scarce, the older women take over. They dig for roots, or tubers, which are highly nutritious and can be found year round. This source of food is hard to find and difficult to get. One of the favored roots is buried deep in rocky soil, and it takes a lot of muscle to dig it up and pull it out. This is something the Hadza children cannot do, but their mothers and grandmothers can. When a newborn comes into the picture, mothers, however, spend more time nursing. That's when Grandma's foraging expertise becomes critical to the survival of her weaned grandchildren.

The GMH theorizes that *grandmother* increases the number of children her daughters can have, thus increasing the chances her genes are passed on. If daughters can depend on grandma to feed younger children, then they can wean current newborns sooner and have another baby. More babies mean more genes going to the next generation, and in this case, more selection for healthier long-lived postmenopausal grandmothers. The longer grandma is capable of foraging—that is, the longer she lives—the more grandchildren she'll have, and the better chances for their survival. In this way the GMH explains why we live so much longer after we lose our fertility compared to our great ape relatives.

So the longer our primitive female ancestors lived without reproducing, the more children her daughters had, and the better chances these grandchildren had for survival. These progeny then passed along these long-living genes, right along with the early infertility genes. This is reproductive altruism at it's best. An older woman not only gives up her own reproduction to avoid death in childbirth so she can continue to nurture her growing infant, toddlers, and preteens, but she also eventually takes care of her daughters and *their* children. This theory celebrates menopause as a milestone, a crucial step in the survival of the family, which may also be the missing link that separates us from the apes at the local zoo!

The Slowing Clock as a Non-adaptive Artifact of Aging

This is the other camp. There is a very strong contingent of evolutionary biologists and anthropologists who believe our sudden decline in fertility and eventual menopause had nothing do with natural selection, and therefore is not an adaptation. This theory lacks a catchy title, and doesn't evoke a warm fuzzy grandmother image, however, its implications are nevertheless equally profound.

Oops What's This? Let's Call It Menopause!

So the question is, if our abbreviated biological clocks are not an adaptation, if this deadline for childbearing doesn't have an important purpose, then why does it exist? The answer according to the non-adaptive camp is that it exists only because we are living longer than ever before. This side argues that throughout prehistoric times, when evolution was in full swing among our hominid ancestors, people rarely made it to 30 or 40, let alone 50 years old. Therefore, what we now anticipate as menopause escaped selection pressure altogether because women, for the most part, were already dead before it could happen. The rare woman who managed to avoid disease, and/or predators, and lived a little longer, gained nothing by doing so in terms of her genetic legacy.

Essentially, this camp believes, menopause is a relatively new physiological phenomenon, simply a consequence of aging well. It has been likened to other diseases of aging, such as Alzheimer's disease or even certain cancers such as prostate cancer. We are seeing these diseases only because we are living longer. In the distant past, natural selection could not do away with the genes that predispose people to these disorders, because nobody lived long enough to have them. In this manner, the vast majority of our ancient female relatives died in advance of experiencing menopause, so there was no way to select for genes having anything to do with it—hence, genes that cause our reproductive systems to wind down persisted throughout time.

A study published in the journal *Nature* provides a foundation for this theory. Evolutionary biologists at both the University of Minnesota and Brown University studied two species with close female social bonds, and whose elderly females help with grandchildren. Both the African lion and the olive baboon have similar characteristics when it comes to lifespan and reproduction. Researchers looked for evidence of menopause as an adaptation, as well as signs that baboon and lion grandmothers benefited their offspring or their grandchildren.

In the baboons, maternity rate remains constant from age 6, when puberty begins, until age 21, when it starts to decrease; fertility drops substantially at age 23, and then ceases altogether at age 24. Interestingly, baboon infant survival rate also drops, and miscarriage rates rise beginning at age 21. Baboon mothers are instrumental in determining their daughter's rank within the troop's hierarchy, and they also groom and look after their grandchildren.

Though it is more difficult to track cycling in lions and there is less data, they show a similar pattern. Their clocks, however, run a little quicker; reproduction begins at age 3 and remains constant until age 13. When lionesses hit 14, fertility takes a sharp dive. The average number of cubs per litter drops from two and a half to one; and the number of litters per year is reduced. When a lion reaches 17, she no longer reproduces at all. Female lions also have a strong social bond. Related female lions help each other defend their pride's territory; they hunt together and will raise cubs communally; grandma lions even nurse their daughters' cubs.

However, the researchers found no evidence that curtailing reproduction was any sort of adaptation, nor did they see any signs resembling the tenets of the GMH. Study author Craig Packer writes regarding the GMH: "...[N]either the survival of grandchildren nor the reproductive performance of adult daughters is improved in the predicted manner." In fact, the study revealed an opposite effect in lions. "Lion cubs only show higher survival when their grandmothers are reproductively active," writes Packer. That is to say, elderly female lions would suckle their grandchildren only while still mothering and tending to their own cubs. So, in this instance, halting reproduction *reduces* grandma lion's ability to help with the grandchildren.

The research also showed there was no increased risk in pregnancy or childbirth to any of the females who happened to live closer to the upper ends of their expected reproductive life span. Packer's team found no evidence that mortality associated with reproduction, increased with age. In the study groups, no female baboon lived beyond age 28, and no female lion beyond age 18. Most animals died before they ever experienced a decline in reproduction; only a few survived long enough to spend any time living without reproducing. Those that did reproduce at an advanced age had a very short life expectancy thereafter. Researchers also calculated that continuous breeding would leave 0.24 percent more baboon offspring and 0.15 percent more lion offspring than typical females. They concluded, in terms of evolution, it would not be worth it for these animals to keep reproducing to the bitter end.

However, on second glance, Packer noted a compelling distinction between the time of the female's last births and the time of their deaths. When baboons' fertility begins to decline at age 21, they have another five years of life expectancy. This is just enough time to rear any last offspring. Baboons need about two years to care for their offspring; baboon babies are much more likely to die if they are orphaned before they reach 2 years old. Any offspring born much after mother baboon is 21 will have a good chance of being orphaned too early to make it on its own.

With lions, cubs need their mothers for the first year of life, after which they have a better chance of surviving on their own. As noted earlier, once a lion mother reaches 14, her fertility drops, but what is striking is that she has approximately 1.8 years left to live—a perfect window of time to rear her last offspring. Packer suggests this mechanism could have also been at work in ancestral humans. If a woman actually lived long enough to experience a decline in fertility at around age 40, she could then expect to make it into her 50s; precisely the amount of time that seems to correspond to the number of years necessary to ensure survival of her last child. According to the non-adaptive theory, this could be the reason human females evolved a menopause at about the same age: it was just enough time to rear the last offspring, and right about when they could expect to die.

Remember this is all theory, but given observations in other mammals, Packer says, "Prolonged infant dependency seems sufficient to account for a midlife menopause in human females." He also suggests infant dependency can explain why women lose their reproductive capacity much sooner and more suddenly than men—most mammals depend on their mothers far more for their survival than they do on their fathers. So rather than some grand design for grandmothers to help with the grandchildren, Packer and others believe the clock was structured right along with what evolution intended for our lifespan. It gave us just enough time before our bodies gave out to kick the last one out of the hut. That way our genetic heritage would be preserved in our children, rather than leaving orphans that couldn't survive on their own.

Why Can't They All Just Get Along?

As I said, there isn't much these two camps agree on. Those who believe good grandmothers forced evolution to favor an early loss of fertility, plus a very lengthy menopausal life, are convinced there is no other explanation. Those who adhere to the non-adaptive reasoning are just as adamant that menopause has no value other than a sign that life is nearly over (and from the standpoint of our earliest relatives, it was). From a purely objective and, admittedly, layperson's perspective, the GMH makes us all feel good about our fertility decline and menopausal life—it means we are supposed to go through it so we can help our grandchildren. It also may explain (if you believe

70

early humans had a lifespan near what it is today) perhaps why we live so long after we go through this change. The non-adaptive theory makes us cringe. What? Suddenly losing fertility is the first sign of our bodies turning straight downhill? That's not a very pleasant thought, especially if it starts right on time at age 41, or sooner. But, that said, it's important to clear the dust a little, put emotions aside, and understand at least a few of the arguments on each side to be able to come to your own conclusion.

Here's What They Have to Say

We started out talking about the adaptation theory and the dangers of childbirth driving the evolutionary system, but the other side believes that at the upper end of the lifespan, which tended to be the end of reproduction, childbirth was not dangerous for women. This is difficult to discern because many women in their 40s give birth without any problem, and many do not. I likely would have been dead at age 40, and my son never born, had I not had the option for a C-section. After 36 hours of labor with the highest dose of labor-inducing drugs, my cervix never made it to the requisite diameter. But many women the same age sail through natural childbirth.

David Keefe, M.D., is unwavering in his belief that the clock is an adaptation based on reproductive altruism; it exists to avoid difficult childbirth, so mothers will be around for the children they already have. Keefe says, "Reproduction is toxic. It could kill you! If you are laying eggs, that's different, but picture yourself in 1000 B.C. delivering a baby in the Alps—it's dangerous. If you start to hemorrhage, you're dead—and now you've left orphans. What's the impact of that?" He says the other camp focuses on the age of menopause too much. "We're not talking about menopause; what we're talking about is something that happens 15 to 20 years before menopause." He believes most women did live past the age of 30 when fertility begins its decline, and, to him, that makes a difference. "If there is a subset of women that was making it to their 30s and 40s, they conferred adaptive value on their offspring—by being around," he insists.

Which brings me to a key difference between both camps. Proponents of the GMH claim the ancient lifespan records are inaccurate. Hawkes agrees with Keefe in that Stone Age women did make it past age 30. She says archeological findings, which purport to estimate lifespan, can be erroneous. This side also believes the record is slanted somewhat by the substantial infant and childhood mortality back in ancient times.

The little information (mind you, this isn't a book about evolution) I dug up showed that a group of Neanderthals found buried in the Middle East lived to ages 24, 36, 40, and 41. Another later group living during the Bronze Age, about 2,000 to 700 B.C., died at ages 3, 6, 8, 9, 30, 40, and 45. If these are correct, then it appears many children died at a young age, and some women probably did make it to be a grandmother.

Those on the non-adaptive side, however, argue that the limited record is probably as accurate as it can possibly be—it's just that not enough of our ancestors lived to see grandmotherhood, and if they did, they certainly didn't live long enough to make a difference in the survival of their grandchildren. The previous example shows many children likely died despite the grandmothers that might have been around.

Although, Hawkes, and others in the adaptive camp, may be correct in claiming the lifespan records are skewed by the large numbers of babies and children that died, it appears unlikely that given the dangers of living B.C., and even up until the antibiotic revolution, that women lived much beyond menopause. In fact, it's no secret that only in the last century has the average expectancy increased substantially. This seems to be an indication that the non-adaptive camp may have an edge. (There will be more discussion about lifespan in Chapter 8.)

Regardless of which side is correct on lifespan, both sides agree that we humans do live quite a long time without reproducing any further offspring of our own. The GMH says we forfeit our own reproduction so we can become grandmothers and can help with the grandkids. The other side says that the discrepancy may exist so mothers can live just long enough to rear their last child, and any living beyond that is an artifact of modern society and modern medicine only.

Adherents to the GMH also assume early humans had a number of surviving children. But Packer says they were lucky if each individual had just two. "...[T]hat means on average, you're going to have a quarter of mothers who would not have any daughters at all; they'd have sons." He challenges the idea of the GMH because, according to his calculations, there would be a good portion of grandmothers without daughters to look after.

Still, having infertile grandmothers around was important for helping mothers bear more children, feeding those children, and even allowing families, perhaps entire colonies, to move around to new locations. With a troop of hardworking older women able to forage for foods difficult to find and extract, these early ancestors became mobile, rather than remaining limited to staying where the pickings would be easy enough for children to retrieve on their own. The Hadza tribe has provided a good example of this.

However, Packer's camp counters, that if the GMH is valid, there should be some evidence in other long-lived mammals, though so far none has been found. He suggests the Hadza case may not extend to all of human evolution. The Hadza grandmothers may have been an exception, or perhaps simply keeping busy, proposes Packer. "If you have a woman who happens to still be alive who no longer is capable of child rearing herself, what the hell else is there for her to do? Of course she'll look after her grandchildren."

As I'm sure you can appreciate, much more research must be done before there can possibly be consensus on exactly how our relentless biological clock evolved, or if it evolved at all.

Nature Is Robbing Women of Nurture

Most people, even the anthropologists and evolutionary biologists, would agree this reproductive program is outdated in today's civilized, technological society. More and more women are running up against this clock, trying to have children when much to their surprise, they are at the end of the reproductive road. They are essentially looking over that proverbial fertility cliff. These women often have no children, so whether you support the reproductive altruism theory, the GMH, or non-adaptive theory, they're all useless because they only make sense if you already have children. It doesn't matter which one has more merit, or might even be exactly correct, if you look at it from the perspective of millennium women who want to start their families after 35 or 40. In addition, it's obvious this clock is no longer needed, because women now face no greater danger in childbirth at age 50 than they do at 20. Twentieth century medicine has removed that selective pressure entirely. So, if this early reproductive decline was a marvelous adaptation at one time, the rationale for it no longer exists.

Whatever mechanism the forces of nature worked out thousands, if not millions, of years ago to help us pass on our genes—it is no longer effective. How can it be if we now use contraception, postpone children, and decide to *start* our families when our ancestors were about to retire their ovaries for the good of the children they already had, and/or their little grandkids? Many contemporary women trying to have children despite a slowing clock have no children, and will therefore never have grandchildren! This is not what Mother Nature intended when she decided the timing of this clock was a good idea.

Let's also remember that when our clock was under evolutionary construction, women started having children as soon as they became fertile—say age 14 or 15. This practice remained fairly constant until relatively recent history. When William Shakespeare wrote *Romeo and Juliet* in 1595 or 1596, society was just beginning to rethink the idea of very young teenagers getting married. The line mentioning Juliet's age: "…hath not seen the change of fourteen years," reminds us just how young was slightly too young in late 16th century England.

It wasn't until the mid-20th century when women began demanding equality in education, and more recently the workforce, that delaying marriage and childbirth became the norm. Couple this with the phenomenon of unprecedented health and lifespan for women, and it's no wonder we want, and expect, we can have children later in life. Unfortunately, the clock, which for one reason or another has been locked up in our genes throughout the ages, is not about to accommodate us. This is a problem.

It is estimated that in the United States, between a third and a half of all successful career women have no children. According to Sylvia Ann Hewlett, in an article for the *Harvard Business Review*, these include business executives, doctors, lawyers, and academics who are anywhere from 41 to 55 years old. The sad thing is, the vast majority of them did not choose to be childless—in fact, they would love to have children. Hewlett conducted a nationwide survey to document the scope of the problem; the results were featured in her book, *Creating a Life: Professional Women and the Quest for Children* (Miramax, 2002).

74

Hewlett says the findings are both "startling—and troubling. They make it clear that, for many women, the brutal demands of ambitious careers, the asymmetries of male-female relationships, and the difficulties of bearing children late in life conspire to crowd out the possibility of having children." Also just for the record, in today's society, the decade that women (and men) require to build a successful career, whether it involves advanced degrees, climbing the corporate ladder, or launching a business, completely overlaps with the best time to start a family. It's no wonder they wait. But there is a price. This clock essentially denies many women equality in career building, or family building—a dilemma many young ambitious men never have to face. As one observer put it, there are many ways *off* the career highway, but few ways back on.

Un-natural Selection?

Given the sad state of family affairs for high-achieving women, I asked Craig Packer, who is (whether or not you agree with his take on the origins of the human reproductive clock) a leading evolutionary biologist, what, if anything, this lack of genetic heritage might mean for the future. I wondered if so many evidently bright, creative, ambitious, and therefore successful women, are unable to pass on their genes, could that spell trouble for our species, or at least society? Packer answered, "That's scary. If the women who are most likely to get caught short by delaying their reproduction have a genetic constitution whereby they're more independent, they're more intelligent, they're more curious, or whatever, then this is really a sad thing on a population level." However, he continued, "If we imagine that it's an accident of their upbringing…that those same characters of intelligence and independence, etc., are found in all women, but not all of them end up on this particular [no children] track, then I wouldn't say there would be any evolutionary shift at all." He tends to believe the latter is true, but what if the trend continues, and more women who are at the upper percentiles for characteristics such as intelligence, creativity, and drive to make a difference, are not passing on these much-valued traits to the extent they would have been? Marcelle Cedars, M.D., reproductive endocrinologist and researcher, believes we should be concerned. "You are losing a lot of your brain power for the future if these women don't have children. If you're trying to save your strong gene pool, that's not what we're doing in this country. That seems to never get discussed." You can draw your own conclusions.

Another more immediate result of this clash between the clock and social trends is the emotional toll it takes on women and families. Women who miss the deadline for having their own genetic children feel a tremendous amount of regret, and often spend months if not years grieving the loss of the children they will never have. Those who do manage to have a first child after age 35 or even after 40 may not be able to have another and complete their families. Secondary infertility is rampant among educated, ambitious, professional married women. Though, "only" children generally do fine, it bears mentioning that this antiquated clock exacts a toll on them as well. Many grow up without siblings they would have had, if only women had just a little more time to create their families.

How to Fix It

Contrary to popular belief, there are ways to deal with our childbearing deadline. None are especially easy. Though it seems at this point in time, we really have no choice but to take action if we want to get an education, build a career, *and* have a family.

The Extra-Long-Term Plan

In the interest of full disclosure, the clock itself could be on the verge of changing. In the words, again, of Craig Packer, "...[I]f conditions have been favoring later reproduction, for all kinds of economic reasons, and there's a genetic variance in how late people can reproduce, I would certainly predict that the age of menopause [and fertility decline] gets later and later through evolutionary time." Packer adds in a nonchalant tone, "It's formidable...you're speaking 10s of generations at the least."

So eventually natural selection may indeed mold our clocks to better suit the changing needs of our society. It's nice to know that if the current trends continue, Mother Nature could turn things around for future generations, but for you, and for my daughter, and for several future generations, other changes must occur first. If we are successful in creating these changes, perhaps Mother Nature can move on to other pressing tasks.

Attitude Adjustment

For the foreseeable future, your clock is *your* clock. It is not going to change so that you can plan to have children when you decide the time is right. As you will see in Chapter 4, there are ways to estimate your individual clock, and ways to keep it in tip-top shape, but it is still on it's own timetable, and will eventually systematically decline. You must make plans accordingly, and in order to do this, you have to adjust any fantasies of having control over when the best time is for you to start and complete your family. Make no mistake your clock determines that. Either you adjust to it, or you may lose your chance of having your own genetic children.

After adjusting your thinking towards living with this uncontrollable time frame for children, it would be highly advisable for you to make a further attitude modification. This is probably the more difficult of the two: Children are absolutely wonderful. I'm not just saying that because I have one, and one on the way. There is nothing more fulfilling and joyous in life than raising a child. In all my years of TV reporting—going where the action is; reporting live from major crime scenes; covering major disasters, including Ground Zero; interviewing celebrities and top political figures; even covering the president many times—none of it, and I mean combine it all together, and none of it comes close to watching that first step, or more recently his first run down a ski slope. I'm not trying to be corny; I never would have believed it either, but it happens to be true. Also, understand that I absolutely loved my career. It's all I ever wanted to do, and I did it for a long time. Having a child is better.

The take-home message is, no matter how much of a charge you get out of your career, a child, without even trying, can thrill you beyond your wildest dreams. Children add a dimension to your life that you can't even imagine until you have them. Even if a child isn't precisely planned for the moment you get the news, you may be surprised at how much better your life becomes. I realize this is an arduous shift to make, given we are so programmed from an early age that getting pregnant and having a child is not a good thing. And granted, in our teens, and much of our 20s, if we have no means to support a child, this program serves us well. However, once we reach our late 20s, this agenda really should change. This is the time to start planning, one way or another, for children, if you think you want them.

It's important to remember, this is an opportunity in life you don't want to miss—and you very easily could if you fail to adjust your thinking and allow your clock to tick away rather than take some action. If you are highly motivated, see the sections on egg freezing on pages 160–166.

Once you have made your decision, you may want to convince your spouse if you are married. (If you are not, see Chapter 4, step 2, on how best to deal with boyfriends.) Men are even more programmed than women. Many women I've talked to say their husbands wanted to wait to have children. Wait for what? To take another vacation? To save a few more bucks? If you are married to a great guy, have a good marriage, and want children, don't wait—you won't regret it.

Bring Your New Attitude to Work

If you are reading this you are likely planning a career, building one, or maintaining one. Some careers are more demanding than others. I chose a ridiculous career to combine with having a family. In the news business, producers, executive producers, and news directors generally have zero regard for family. It is a very insular culture, also very youth-oriented. The newsroom is all that matters, it is your first home, and those with whom you work are your family members, and this family comes together day after day to deal with crisis after crisis after crisis. Every one of these crises, or news stories, happens when it happens. There is no such thing as a "work day." As a reporter, I would start my days generally at the same time, although many mornings began with the telephone ringing and a request to come in early, rather than an alarm clock. And there was no telling when a day would end. I wish I had a nickel for every time I heard these words following my 6 o'clock live shot: "Hi Cara, we'd like you stay and do a live shot for the 11. We don't have another reporter to come out there, you are it." Of course, I also worked nights, weekends, and early mornings—a start time of 3 o'clock in the morning.

A job doesn't get more incompatible to family life than TV reporting. I know more women TV reporters who do not have children than do. Most of those without children either want or wanted them. Still, it is possible to have just about any career you desire *and* have a family. It simply takes effort and an awareness to be able to beat the clock. It helps to work in a field or for a company that values family, or at the very least, work for a boss who values you and understands what a family is about. Don't expect that a woman who has a child will be any more compassionate than a woman without one.

I'm not going to sugarcoat the difficulties. Remaining in an extremely demanding career is difficult when you start your family. I was up for a promotion at my station when I was pregnant with my son. I remember hiding it as long as possible, then finally sitting down and telling my boss. She seemed very happy for me, and I was relieved. However, I did not get the job. Someone who wasn't pregnant, and five years hence still has no kids, got the position. The day after my son was born, I received a call from a friend at the same TV station who told me another position was coming available. I wobbled down the hospital hallway in agony from the incision of my C-section to call this same boss. I remember clearly saying, "I want this position. Don't count me out because I just had a child." That position went to a guy 15 years younger than me. A year or so later, that boss, who had one child, received a promotion, and was replaced. The new woman, who had no children, told me she would promote me in a heartbeat if she had a position, but given the economic downturn, it was unlikely there would be any in the foreseeable future. She was right, there haven't been any since.

The moral of this story for younger women: it helps to choose a field that is more compatible to family life; a bit of effort to explore a variety of careers will pay off. Also, if you are on the corporate track, which according to Hewlett is one of the most difficult for families, try researching companies with solid and proven family-friendly policies. Lists of these companies are available annually, and companies vie to get on them. *Working Mother* magazine has one of the most popular lists.

However, if you are like me, and you simply have to work in an extremely competitive, demanding field, or you find yourself in a company where few people have children, and the family-friendly waters haven't been tested, I would highly recommend you remind yourself how valuable you are to that company, and celebrate the fact that you are starting your family. Your desire to have a family shouldn't be doom and gloom for your career; it should be a major milestone in your life that your boss and coworkers will cheer. In a competitive environment, you simply do what you have to do to survive. It will mean less time with your child or children, but you make it work, any way you can.

If it's not a matter of job or no job, then when the time comes, think about exploring some other options, such as job sharing, flexible hours, or working at home one or two days a week, to avoid the commute. Commuting can be a monumental waste of time whether you have a family or not. If you can get more work done from home just by avoiding a long commute, tell your boss, do a trial run, and show her the results. Face-time isn't all that important when you get the work done in half the time. And you will get more work done—there are many more distractions in an office than there are at home.

The more women who decide to stay in the workforce, carve out a workable niche, and demand that their career not suffer, the better off all of us will be. We cannot expect to be workaholics when we have children and a household to maintain. If you have succeeded to some extent in your position and career, it is possible to continue in that career. This is also the only way corporate America will change the persistent negative attitudes towards working mothers. Even in companies that tout their family-friendly polices, Hewlett says, "...[A] widespread belief in business is that a woman who allows herself to be accommodated on the family front is no longer choosing to be a serious contender." She insists that top management must work hard to deprogram this kind of thinking in the corporate culture. The more women insist on remaining serious contenders while growing families, the sooner managers and top executives will get the message. Even though this may seem like a long, difficult process, it's still easier and more efficient than depending on technology, or waiting for Mother Nature to nudge our biological clocks into giving us extra time.

Science, Science, Science

Eventually, science will give us more flexibility in family building. Anyone affiliated with the infertility field is well aware of the need for such advances, though research is hardly a funding priority. Much of this work is privately funded, and therefore maintains an incredibly sluggish pace. The hottest research into fixing this clock dilemma that so many women now face is egg freezing. Several groups are working relentlessly toward improving techniques for submerging mature eggs into a deep freeze without damaging their delicate internal structures. Eventually, any woman will be able to freeze some eggs at an early age, to use later, if life circumstances unfold in a way that the clock

80

becomes a problem. This technology is already available at a few clinics, though poised to expand. Other groups are freezing immature egg tissue, with the idea of transplanting it later, then harvesting mature eggs from it to use for in vitro fertilization. (You will find a comprehensive look at all of these technologies in Chapter 7.)

However, less is being done to determine how to protect eggs while they are still inside our ovaries so they might maintain greater numbers and remain viable for much longer. Many believe there should be a way to halt this inevitable fertility decline, but more time and energy must be invested toward that end.

Another interesting research project that is currently under consideration for funding is the first ever controlled investigation into the genetics of aging and reproduction in baboons. Craig Packer, Ph.D., and David Keefe admit to often heated debates about the origin of reproductive decline and menopause, but they hope to collaborate on this long-term project, which they believe will lead to a discovery of genetic markers that signal premature aging, including early reproductive decline and menopause in individuals. Such markers could direct further research into treatments that could target precisely those areas, which can slow down the process. Both researchers believe the unprecedented investigation would yield a tremendous amount of scientific knowledge about aging and menopause, though neither is convinced it will be funded.

Women should be aware of this struggling research, and demand more of it. Let your voice be heard in this debate—this is a major issue in reproductive endocrinology circles, but few others realize what is going on. Legislators and regulators must hear from women and women's advocacy groups, not just the doctors and their organizations that are working in the field. If we want these future options, we have to make it known. The more voices, the better the chances of getting funding, and the closer we might be to having more control over our biological clocks.

10 STEPS THAT WILL INCREASE YOUR FERTILITY POTENTIAL

4.

I wish I had known. I would have planned better and done things differently. I definitely would have taken an FSH test if I had known it existed. I've had four miscarriages in the last two years. I don't know what to do.

—Sandy, age 38

I took an FSH test and found out I might still be fertile! I can't believe it. It took me so long to find the right man, and now we might be able to have a child together. I've checked my cycle and we're going to start trying right away.

—Nancy, age 43

Uncertain Expectations

Nearly every girl who has ever played with a doll thinks she will grow up to be a mommy. It's part of the order of life. But often, as she matures and begins thinking about other ambitions, having children becomes a given, a much-easier-to-accomplish goal, and perhaps less of a priority. It is on the "to do" list, but is placed behind academic and professional achievements.

I was one of those girls. I knew I wanted children, but during my mid- to late 20s when boyfriends were cast aside like worn shoes, I had much more important things to do. A few years later, in my early 30s, I found myself ready to get married and start a family. There was only one problem: now the man in my life had better things to do. That heartbreak brought me into my late 30s, when the ticking of my clock had become more of a clanging. Still, even at 39, when the home pregnancy test read positive, I thought, "Oh, no! This isn't the right time." Little did I know it was the perfect time, and it would likely be the only time.

According to Ellen Glazer, an infertility counselor and author of several books on infertility including *The Long-Awaited Stork: A Guide to Parenting After Infertility* (Jossey-Bass, 1998), this change in attitude happened sometime during the 1970s and 80s when the women's movement was in full swing. "I finished high school in the mid-60s and I know I left believing I had until I was 30 to have children," she says. "In those days, anyone who gave birth over 30 was called a 'geriatric mother.'" The following generations of women found new power and believed they could do anything, including have children well into their 30s and 40s. "I think the women's movement may have prompted people to extend the notion of a geriatric mother a bit too far," Glazer adds.

Of course, if you throw all the advances in reproductive medicine into the mix of messages our generation received, it's no wonder we thought we could do it all, whenever we wanted. Still, the point remains that it is difficult to say when having children should become a priority. It is certainly unrealistic to simply say, "Have your children before age 30." Today many women, in particular college-educated professional women, don't even begin to think about having children until they are 30.

Here's the problem: while we are searching and wondering if the time is right, we haven't any idea what the approximate time is on our biological clocks; we have no idea how many years of fertility we have left. So how on earth can we decide? We generally think, *I'm fertile. As soon as I stop using contraception, I will get pregnant.* But even for women in their early 30s, this isn't necessarily so.

Dr. Pat McShane, director of the Reproductive Science Center just outside Boston, Massachusetts, constantly encounters age-related infertility. "I see new patients every day, and inevitably someone says, 'I wish I had known.'" What if you knew that your fertility was already beginning to decline; that you most likely have just a couple years left? Would that change your decision to wait? What if you finally decide that the time is right, but your partner disagrees? What if there was a way to adjust your cycle? Women are missing a key portion of the information needed to make a major decision!

This chapter changes that. The 10 steps give you the information you need to keep your clock ticking as long as possible; and later you can estimate approximately how long your clock will run. Even if you're not ready to have children, it's important that you start gathering information sooner rather than later. Don't assume you'll get pregnant when you want to. Get to know your reproductive life cycle. Explore your fertility. Calculate your clock.

The Basics

There are several ways to protect your fertility. Some will help avoid medical issues associated with trying to conceive. One fertility doctor I asked about this summed it up, "Condom, condom, condom." Protecting yourself from sexually transmitted diseases can prevent problems conceiving later on. Chlamydia is the most common sexually transmitted infection in the United States. If left untreated, it can spread to the uterus and fallopian tubes and cause pelvic inflammatory disease (PID). This disease can cause infertility by damaging the fallopian tubes, the uterus, as well as surrounding tissue. To make matters worse, this infection usually has no symptoms; only a medical procedure can detect it, so you may not even know you have this problem for many years. In addition to regular condom use, women of reproductive age should have an annual Chlamydia screening test to help avoid problems later. The good news is it can be cured with antibiotics.

Another condition you should be aware of is endometriosis. This disorder is quite common and is characterized by small pieces of endometrial tissue that find their way outside the uterus, into other areas of the body, particularly around the uterus and ovaries. The tissue flares up during the menstrual cycle and causes severe pain. It is estimated that 30 to 40 percent of those with endometriosis go on to suffer infertility. However, it can be treated, though not cured, with proper diagnosis. Fibroids are another problem, these growths, usually benign, can continue to grow unchecked and lead to major health problems including damage to reproductive organs. A single friend just had surgery to remove several fibroids that five years earlier she assumed were just a nuisance. However, many had grown so large that at 39 and childless, her uterus was damaged to the point that it was removed along with the fibroids. She regrets not monitoring them more closely; she still wants children, but will now have to hire a surrogate, as well as potentially an egg donor, or adopt.

Your weight can also affect future fertility. Obesity is a major risk factor for infertility. Being overweight contributes to menstrual disorders and infertility. Obese women undergoing treatment for infertility have a more difficult time getting pregnant than those of normal weight. A sensible diet and exercise program has been shown to reverse this effect. On the other hand, too much dieting and exercising isn't good either—because women who are too thin also risk infertility. Many female athletes (competitive or recreational) stop menstruating due to intense physical training, dieting, and poor nutrition. This may seem like a welcome reprieve, but it is extremely unhealthy. It can cause premature osteoporosis, a higher risk of cardiovascular disease, endometrial cancer, and infertility. However, it can be reversed with an improved diet and a modified training regimen. If you are currently experiencing amenorrhea (a lack of menstrual cycle), you should check with your doctor as soon as possible to avoid severe health problems, including infertility.

Finally, you may have seen articles or media reports that suggest that you "don't wait too long" to have children. But these messages rarely say just how long is too long. Women's lives are much more complicated than they've ever been, and yet this recurring message is so simplistic it borders on meaningless or at the very least, inappropriate. If you are in your early 30s and have been married for a couple of years, "Don't wait too long," might mean something to you. For everybody else, the message is useless! You're left with nothing, no information on what your time frame might be, or what you can do about it.

This chapter is intended to help you understand what you can actually *do* to give yourself as much time as possible with your biological clock, including a way to calculate your deadline for children. The following steps can help anyone avoid wasting time, and buy some of this precious commodity by keeping the gears in your clock as rust-free as possible.

The 10 Steps

These are actions you can take to protect your fertility, potentially preserve it, and at least understand where you are on the biological clock dial. It is not necessary to follow them in order, but you may want to do so for at least the first few.

1. Take an FSH Test

The first thing any 30- or 40-something woman who wants children should do is take an FSH test on day three of her menstrual cycle. You may get some resistance from your doctor at first, but be persistent. Tell your primary care doctor or your gynecologist that you want to know if your fertility is intact. If she tells you, "Don't worry about it, you're fine," tell her you'd like to find out if your FSH is at all elevated. If you still encounter resistance, show her this book, and tell her it's important that you monitor your FSH because you want children and don't want to miss your opportunity. If the discussion goes beyond this point, find another doctor.

Once you have the test result, make sure your doctor understands it completely. Depending on the lab running the test, results and their interpretation may vary; your doctor should be aware of this. See Chapter 1 for a thorough review on how to interpret FSH tests. Essentially, a value under 10 is considered normal, with a fairly good chance of success in treatment with IVF. While no one is yet keeping records of what FSH levels are best for natural conception, what *is* known is that the higher the FSH level, the lower the chances for success with technology. The lower the value, the better, if you are using this test to monitor your fertility and you hope to conceive the old-fashioned way.

If your result is near 10 or above, you shouldn't delay trying to conceive. It is important to get started quickly, so that if there's a problem down the road, you still have hope in treatment. Also, remember that FSH levels are not static; they fluctuate each month. Because the test is a snapshot of your clock on that particular cycle, you may want to monitor every three or six months, or every year depending on your age.

Keep in mind that studies have shown that your fertility is only as good as your *worst* FSH test. If the level is between 10 and 15, your fertility is beginning to decline. You should find a good reproductive endocrinologist. While you are waiting for your appointment, follow the rest of the steps, and start trying to conceive. Any level of 15 or higher usually means that your chances for conception with your own eggs are poor.

2. Talk to Your Partner and Freeze Embryos and Eggs if You Can

If you want a family, then talking with your partner—whether he's a husband, fiancé, or boyfriend—just makes sense. You can decide exactly what to say, but he should be aware that you want children, and he should understand that there is a very definite window of opportunity to do so.

"Once a woman hears the clock ticking, it is very important she share her desire for children with the man in her life. Not doing so can lead both down the road to infertility. The sooner they agree on a time frame to start a family, the better the chances they won't miss their opportunity," says Ellen Glazer, infertility counselor and author.

Your partner should realize that once the window begins closing, it can take a tremendous amount of technology, not to mention emotional pain and physical discomfort, to open it again. If he is at all reluctant, provide the basic information about your biological clock, and then tell him you plan to monitor your FSH. If you've already done the test, tell him the results, and explain what the possible consequences might be if you wait too long. That should be enough to help you reach an understanding with your husband, or help you realize you're with the wrong boyfriend so you don't waste any more time with him.

I've heard so many women say that because their husbands wanted to wait to have children, they put it off. In many cases they regret it.

88

One friend I'll call Betty told me that she resents her husband for insisting they hold off on children. It turns out that in the two years they waited, she lost the ability to have her own genetic children. She is now considering using an egg donor, but the fact that he can still become a genetic father is yet another layer of anger and resentment that she's dealing with. If Betty had known the facts about her biological clock and started monitoring her FSH as soon as she got married, she could have informed her husband and had some hard evidence to present in their conversations. Hers is a heart-wrenching story—she finally met her soul mate at age 38, and two years later their marriage is in peril.

Another friend burst into tears during a conversation with her new husband who wanted to wait at least a year before starting a family. She new she might not have a year; it was now or never for her, whether the marriage worked or not. She got pregnant the same weekend. However, she did experience secondary infertility, and it wasn't until her *fifth* IVF that she conceived her second daughter. The marriage worked out, and her family is complete.

If a man isn't ready for marriage, you can be almost certain he's not ready for children. If you want children and you are in your 30s, it is definitely time to have a talk. Of course you can suggest circumventing marriage, and have your children first. But if you both want a traditional two or so year courtship, one or two year engagement, a year to plan the wedding, a couple of years together, then children— you can do the math. And remember he won't run out of time, *you* will. When you have the discussion, make sure he understands the facts, and let him do the math too. Point out there's little question you will be putting yourself up against the clock.

If you are already married, and your husband insists on waiting and he won't budge, there is something you can do that has proven to work. You and your husband can *freeze embryos*. As long as you are still fertile, the chances of a frozen embryo becoming a baby years down the road are extremely good. Most couples who freeze embryos do so as part of their IVF treatment, that is, they freeze the "leftover" fertilized embryos in case the fresh embryos do not implant or to use them later if they want to try for more children.

Most married women who are fertile and delaying starting their families don't exercise this option because they don't know it exists.

But embryos are frozen every day inside fertility clinics, and women often get pregnant with frozen embryos that have been in cold storage for months or even years. You ought to at least think about this option if you have a long-term partner or husband, and for whatever reason, you can't start your family in your late 20s or early 30s. Don't wait until your clock starts slowing down. Freeze some good embryos while you have the chance.

If you are single and believe you are fertile, but expect to delay having children, you might also consider freezing your eggs. Turn to Chapter 7 as well as the Resource section for details and information on this brand-new (though still considered experimental) option.

3. Get to Know Your Cycle

A normal cycle is 28 days with ovulation occurring between days 12 and 14, on average. If you have intercourse every day, this may not matter, but most couples, especially those over 30 and with busy professional lives, generally need to make sure they are having intercourse on the right days to conceive a baby.

Count the first day of your period as day one if you get a full flow before 5 p.m. Then mark days eight through 15 on the calendar; these are the days you should have intercourse. Make sure there aren't any scheduling conflicts, especially on days 8 through 13. If your cycle is generally

> **!** CAUTION: If you use an ovulation kit and get a positive result in the morning, then try to have sex later that night, you may miss prime time. Remember the egg is viable for only 12 to 24 hours after ovulation. The ovulation kit tells you the approximate window of ovulation, not exactly when it will occur.

shorter or longer than 28 days, you can adjust the time frame back or forward by the number of days less or over 28. For example, if you average 27-day cycles, mark days seven through 14; if you average 30-day cycles, mark days 10 through 17. Normal sperm can live for three days, and if conditions are right may even make it to five days. It is preferable to give plenty of sperm the opportunity to swim through the cervix, then the length of your uterus and into your fallopian tubes where they can come in contact with a mature egg. Fertilization occurs in the ampulla, or the widest segment of the fallopian tube. So if you have intercourse one, two, or three days before ovulation, theoretically, some sperm will arrive early and be ready when a mature egg appears. This is much more art than science, so err on the conservative side, and start having intercourse early and often! If having sex four or five days in a row is difficult, try every other day (on days 8, 10, 12, or on days 9, 11, 13).

It is critical that you check your calendar, understand how ovulation works, and get an approximation of when you ovulate *before* you begin trying to conceive. Each month you have a very small window of opportunity. If your schedule or your husband's conflicts with the critical days, conception won't happen. I checked the calendar the same month we were going to start, and found we couldn't. My husband's schedule was completely out of synch with my cycle. When I was ovulating, he was away working. He was on a two-week rotating schedule, so this presented a formidable challenge. Had I checked a few months earlier, I would have had more months to try to do something about it. I'll never know if it would have made a difference.

4. Adjust Your Cycle With Birth Control Pills if Necessary

I took birth control pills to try to get pregnant. Really, it's true. Hopefully you won't have to do this, but it was a tremendous help to me. If you have a conflict in your schedule, and can't be together during "prime time," you can adjust your cycle. I can't tell you the emotional agony I went through when I was ovulating and my husband was on his ship in the middle of the Gulf of Mexico. One doctor's answer to this problem was to freeze his sperm and do IUIs (intrauterine insemination) to the tune of $1,300 each month. We tried this method twice, and it didn't work. Finally, months later, while pursuing a story on infertility, I met with another doctor. He immediately responded to my quandary, "Oh that's an easy fix. You just use birth control pills. We do it all the time." Here is the method he gave me: The day you start your period, start taking birth control pills. You keep taking the pills until a couple of days before you want your next cycle/period to start. When you stop the pills, you'll get your period within a few days, starting a new cycle. Then you can start counting the days to ovulation again. You should decide in advance approximately when you want ovulation to occur, making sure you and your husband will be together, then count backward 12 or so days to when your period should start, and you stop the pills a couple of days before that.

It worked for me. I got pregnant twice using this method. (Unfortunately, both ended in miscarriages.) There is also evidence that the chances for pregnancy are greater if you use birth control pills during the cycle immediately prior to trying to conceive. Several studies have shown that pregnancy rates rise when women take the birth control pill prior to undergoing IVF treatment. One published in the medical journal *Fertility and Sterility* revealed that using birth control pills for one month prior to IVF enhances pregnancy rates in the following two cycles. In this study, the pregnancy rate doubled! The authors were unable to pinpoint the reason; however, they suggest anovulation, or the lack of ovulation due to the pills, may allow the ovaries some "quiet time," providing better conditions for developing healthier eggs in the following months.

5. Quit Smoking and Lessen Your Exposure to Secondhand Smoke

If you are smoking as you are reading, put the cigarette out. If you have a pack of cigarettes in your pocketbook, throw it out. If you don't have children yet, and you think you may want them, this is the step you must take if you are to keep your fertility at its highest potential. There is little question given the research on this topic that smoking will cause an earlier menopause, and therefore an earlier decline in fertility.

So, put this warning on the side of your cigarette pack: *Smoking causes infertility*. Some might argue that it is a natural process, it just happens sooner. However, if you want a child at 37, and you can't because your eggs are already in poor shape, but you were *supposed* to lose that capacity at say 40, that's infertility. Studies show, and most reproductive endocrinologists agree, that smoking can cause a one to four year deficit in your fertility. This is based on research showing the age of menopause for smokers vs. non-smokers; also the findings are supported by what fertility specialists see in clinics when comparing rates of pregnancy for those who smoke vs. those who don't. Clinics report it takes nearly twice as many IVF tries for smokers to conceive than non-smokers, and in older women, the negative effects are even more pronounced, often to such a degree that technology cannot help achieve a pregnancy.

An interesting study put out by the College of Physicians and Surgeons at Columbia University in New York actually analyzed the ovaries of premenopausal women ages 35 to 54 who underwent hysterectomies. The reason for the hysterectomies had nothing to do with their ovaries, which were normal. Researchers wanted to compare the actual number of follicles (the sacs that contain eggs) in the ovaries of smokers vs. non-smokers. What they found was striking. Both current and ex-smokers had follicle counts that were approximately half that of those who never smoked. They also found no difference between follicle counts in women who smoked for less or more than 15 years and those who smoked for less or more than seven years. These findings reflect previous work that has shown a 40-percent increased risk of menopause before age *40* in current or ex-smokers.

The American Society for Reproductive Medicine warns in a patient fact sheet, "Smoking appears to accelerate the loss of eggs and reproductive function and may advance the time of menopause by several years." Researchers believe this is due to the toxins in cigarette smoke and the fact that eggs in the ovaries appear to be very susceptible to their effects. Massachusetts General Hospital researcher Jonathan Tilly, Ph.D., and his team showed that chemicals called polycyclic aromatic hydrocarbons (PAHs) found in cigarette smoke attach to the insides of egg cells. This attachment triggers a gene that initiates a kind of molecular suicide command, and the egg cell dies. Tilly showed this initially in mice, but then transplanted human ovarian tissue including eggs under the skin of mice and exposed them to the same PAHs. The human eggs died exactly the same way the mouse eggs died.

There's no doubt that smoking can outright kill your precious eggs, but other research also shows it can cause more subtle abnormalities in the chromosomes inside eggs. So, even an egg that is capable of being fertilized may be unable to produce a viable fetus. Smoking is therefore strongly associated with a higher risk of miscarriage. In a Canadian study of women undergoing IVF, researchers found the number of chromosomal abnormalities in eggs correlated with the number of cigarettes smoked—suggesting that the eggs of smokers could not divide properly and therefore could not produce a viable pregnancy.

Other studies looked at cotinine (by-product of nicotine) levels in the follicular fluid (fluid inside the follicle that contains the egg). Results showed 100 percent of smokers had cotinine in their follicular fluid, and the more the women smoked, the higher the continine level was. Researchers also found that 100 percent of women who had been exposed to passive cigarette smoke in the home, also contained this major metabolite of nicotine, though in lower concentrations. So if you don't smoke but live with a smoker, and have for some time, you might be losing eggs anyway.

The American Society of Reproductive Medicine (ASRM) also warns that the impact of passive smoking, or secondhand smoke, is only slightly less than for active smoking. Tilly agrees it's best to stay away from tobacco smoke. "I think it could be a problem, simply because the chemicals are there and we know what the chemicals do when we put them into either human or mouse ovaries, they kill eggs."

So quit, or don't start, and stay away from secondhand smoke as much as possible.

6. Reduce Your Exposure to Environmental Toxins

You've no doubt heard the latest on pesticides or other industrial toxins and their effect on *sperm* count. These reports are fairly common—and it's easy to understand why. It's extremely straightforward to do studies regarding male fertility. You take a group of men who may work or live in an area with a particular risk of a certain exposure and you send them to the bathroom with a cup in hand, once, twice, 10 times over whatever period of time you are researching, and then snap on your microscope and start counting. Easy. It's made even simpler when using male mice: you can directly expose them to toxins, and you don't even need a cup!

It's a little different when trying to assess the effects of environmental toxins on eggs inside ovaries, inside living, breathing women. It makes biologic sense that given what we know about the more targeted and constant exposure of toxins through cigarette smoke that eggs would also be susceptible to other environmental exposures. Though, you might think eggs would be protected given they are deep within the body and kind of hermetically sealed, wrapped up like your mother's wedding gown in the attic, compared to sperm that is stored within millimeters of the outside environment. But some of these toxins can get past the ovaries' protective seal. These toxins are lipophilic, meaning they simply diffuse to the fat tissue that surrounds the egg. One such toxin is arsenic, a naturally occurring heavy metal. David Keefe published two studies regarding the impact arsenic may have on egg viability. "Arsenic has a very potent effect. It gets into eggs then slips into their mitochondria where the toxin promotes reactive oxygen release and shortens telomeres. This essentially ages the egg, rendering it unable to produce a viable fetus," says Keefe.

In these animal studies, small amounts of arsenic were used in order to detect subtle effects on cells. The results showed that more than 60 percent of the eggs were abnormal after exposure to arsenic. These eggs could not divide properly and were either incapable of being fertilized, or had trouble staying alive if they did fertilize.

Okay, I know what you are thinking, *Arsenic? Where would I be exposed to arsenic?* The answer is just about anywhere including your drinking water, depending on where you live. Because arsenic is a naturally occurring mineral found in rocks and soil, it can be found in water. Due to mounting health concerns, the Environmental Protection Agency (EPA) is dropping the safe limit for arsenic from 50 μg/L (micrograms per liter) to 10 μg/L. In areas of the Southwest where arsenic naturally occurs in higher concentrations in the environment, it has been detected at more than 50 μg/L in groundwater supplies. According to the U.S. Geological Survey (USGS), arsenic concentrations likely to exceed the new safe limit are found in upwards of 35 percent of small public water supply systems in the United States. The USGS also notes that homeowners with private wells, which are not regulated, could be drinking water that exceeds the new standard for arsenic. All public water systems must comply with these new limits by January 2006.

Arsenic is also found in the groundwater due to human activities such as agricultural applications, mining, and smelting. It is also a top contaminant at many U.S. Superfund sites. However, if you were to come in contact with arsenic, it most likely would be in your own backyard. For decades, arsenic has been used to heat-pressurize wood used for construction. It is estimated this wood has been used to build more than 90 percent of all outdoor wooden structures in the United

States. So if you have a backyard deck, porch, or anything made of exposed wood, it likely contains arsenic.

Even though the wood is sealed when new, it takes just six months for the sealant to wear off. After that, studies have shown arsenic leaches onto the wood's surface and everywhere around the wood, including the soil beneath it. A consumer group called the Environmental Working Group, in conjunction with the University of North Carolina, found dangerous levels of arsenic in the soil from two out of every five backyards or parks. They also found that the amount of arsenic wiped off a small area of wood, approximately the size of a 4-year-old's hand, usually exceeded the EPA limit for a glass of drinking water.

Bottom line: find out whether you may be overexposed to arsenic, and avoid it if you can. This is a good idea regardless of your future family planning because arsenic is a known carcinogen, with chronic exposure linked to increased risk of cancers of the lung, skin, bladder, and liver. You can buy arsenic testing kits for $20 to $35.

Other environmental toxins are also linked to reproduction problems. The National Institute for Occupational Safety and Health (NIOSH) has made learning about the reproductive effects of toxins a national priority research area. They have a lot of work to do. NIOSH admits that although more than 1,0000 workplace chemicals have shown adverse reproductive effects in animals, most have not been studied in humans; and most of the 4 million other chemical mixtures in commercial use haven't been tested at all.

Make no mistake; we are all exposed to these environmental toxins to some degree. The Centers for Disease Control (CDC) as well as the Mount Sinai School of Medicine in collaboration with the Environmental Working Group (EWG) have begun to actually test people for these contaminants. Both looked at blood and urine samples from average people with no reported significant toxic exposures. The CDC tested nearly 4,000 volunteers and detected 27 potentially toxic substances; the EWG tested nine volunteers, and found a total of 167 pollutants or chemicals in the group.

If you work in a field where you are handling chemicals, solvents, pesticides, or other environmental hazards, take steps to protect yourself and try to limit your exposure. Some toxins are difficult to avoid mostly because they are everywhere or hidden in the food supply.

Heavy metals such as mercury, lead, and cadmium all make their way into the food chain, and all have reproductive effects. The best way to avoid this kind of exposure is to stay away from freshwater fish, where high levels have been detected. This step may also decrease your exposure to PCBs (polychlorinated biphenyls), which have been strongly linked to infertility. In a study of women who ate sport fish from Lake Ontario, researchers from the University at Buffalo, State University of New York, found those who ate the fish for three to six years, at a rate of more than just one fish meal per month, had more difficulty getting pregnant than controls.

Finally, be aware of the environment around you, and do simple things like wash all fruits and vegetables thoroughly, don a face mask when using strong cleansers or solvents such as paint thinners, and take your daily jog at a time other than rush hour if you live in a city, because car exhaust fumes have been shown to damage sperm quality. Nobody knows what it can do to eggs.

7. Make Sure Your Diet Is Rich in Antioxidants

All this means is…eat your fruits and veggies! Though in the interest of full disclosure, there is no direct evidence that says eating a diet high in antioxidants will do wonders for your fertility. But in dozens of interviews, I have yet to find an RE or fertility researcher who says anything other than, "It can't hurt." They all say there's no research specifically pointing to such a recommendation. I came up with only one recent published study that looked at maternal aging and dietary supplementation—in the mouse. The findings showed the antioxidants vitamins C and E had a positive effect. The mice produced more eggs at a later age with both high and low doses of the supplements. The authors caution against comparing this to human effects, but say the results could have "direct" implications for "preventing or delaying maternal age-associated infertility." I will also caution you not to run out and buy megadoses of vitamins C and E based on this one study in mice. More on why this isn't a good idea a bit later. However, the fact that someone designed and carried out this research illustrates this line of investigation is credible, and further study, which is underway, could yield some solid evidence.

In the meantime, it is biologically plausible that just as antioxidants may stem the tide of cell malfunction that leads to cancer, they may also help reduce the deleterious effects of chemicals, toxins, and perhaps even natural aging, in egg cells. Given the overall health benefits to begin with—why wait for the definitive research results? If you are not concerned about the risk of cancer, then keep reading for some basic information that, albeit indirectly, will justify keeping a steady flow of fruits and vegetables in your diet to potentially protect your fertility.

Back in Chapter 2, we took a look at new research on telomere length and its connection to the viability of an egg. As you recall, over time telomeres shorten (bad for eggs!) for a number of reasons. One of them is oxidative damage due to free radicals, which are very unstable oxygen molecules. These free radicals basically chew away on the telomeres, wreaking havoc on eggs. This daily cellular bombardment by free radicals happens throughout the body naturally as we age, and can lead to cancer. Indeed, some research highly suggests that oxidative damage to cells, and the resulting telomere shortening *is* aging. This is because once telomeres shorten enough, cells can no longer divide, and they die. Studies have also shown "oxidation" is one of the principal methods by which toxins and other environmental hazards damage cells, and may lead to cancer. But here's what is important. In some of this research, including Keefe's arsenic work with eggs, researchers show that antioxidants are able to prevent or reverse this damage.

Furthermore, over the past 20 years a cornucopia of evidence has revealed that eating lots of fruits and vegetables is the best way to counteract the destructive work of free radicals. If antioxidants consistently prevent or reverse oxidation damage to cells in a petri dish, and people who eat fruits and vegetables containing high amounts of antioxidants routinely have lowered risks of all kinds of cancers, AND, similarly, the same oxidation process destroys eggs, with antioxidants able to prevent this destruction, then there is only one reasonable thing you can deduce: antioxidants might just help keep eggs healthier longer.

However, don't just start popping vitamin supplements. The vast majority of research thus far on vitamin supplementation containing antioxidants has either shown no effect or proved inconclusive. In fact, some studies on the potent antioxidant beta-carotene given as a supplement have resulted in a rise in lung cancer risk in smokers. Researchers so far haven't figured out why.

For now the best advice is lots of fruits and vegetables, generally at least five servings a day, and less emphasis on the vitamins, especially megadoses, which could have adverse effects, at least when it comes to lung cancer. Speaking of adverse effects, recent research has revealed that it may be best to avoid the fad high-protein, low-carb diets. Researchers revealed at a European medical conference that embryos from mice fed a high-protein diet failed to implant or develop in the uterus more often than those on a more normal diet.

One last note on your fruits and vegetables: the brighter the color, the better. For some reason, dark or brightly colored fruits and vegetables seem to slow the aging process. Blueberries in particular have been shown to actually reverse some symptoms of aging. After feeding elderly rats blueberries every day for several weeks, their balance, coordination, and memory improved. James Joseph, Ph.D., the principal investigator at the U.S. Department of Agriculture Human Nutrition Research Center on Aging at Tufts University, says the effect is likely due to antioxidant capacity, plus some other factor. Interestingly, as soon as Joseph started seeing the results of his own study, he began drinking a blueberry smoothie every day! If blueberries and other colorful fruits and vegetables can work wonders on overall aging and even prevent cancer, it's very possible there could be some positive effect on the biological clock too.

8. Stop or at Least Slow Intake of Caffeine and Alcohol

I used to drink coffee all day long. I'd make a pot first thing in the morning, and drink it until I left for work, sometimes even taking a "go-cup" for the commute. Often, I'd purchase a cup at the TV station's cafeteria before I left on my assignment, and if not, I'd ask my photographer to pull over at the first Dunkin' Donuts or Starbucks I'd see on the road. In fact, I know where every Dunkin' Donuts shop is in greater Boston, and in many parts of New England. I'd also have coffee with lunch, and another fill-up later in the afternoon before I prepared my live report.... You get the picture. *Lots* of caffeine.

As soon as I walked into a fertility clinic, they instantly suggested I stay away from caffeine. Wish I had known! I panicked, and gave up everything that contained caffeine, even chocolate. I checked the labels on soda, and made sure my husband remembered to make decaffeinated coffee for me in the morning. I also turned to tea, and started drinking green tea, because I heard it would help conception. However, a month later after yet another cycle of "trying" failed, I discovered that green tea contains caffeine! Unless the packaging on tea says NO CAFFEINE, it likely contains the substance. If you decide to take this step, you have to become a caffeine detective, because it is hidden in an assortment of foods and drinks—anything that contains either coffee or cocoa, such as hot chocolate, ice cream, cookies, and candy, in addition to a variety of beverages, and over the counter medications.

The science on caffeine is fairly clear. More than two or three cups of coffee per day has been shown in several studies to impair fertility. That is *cups*, as in a standard 8-ounce cup, not a mug, a "grande," or supersize regular. Using coffee as the standard, there are about 100 milligrams of caffeine in one cup of coffee. You can see how it can add up quickly. Though I rarely finished my many cups of coffee during the day, I'm sure I consumed well over a thousand milligrams of caffeine per day.

Much of the research on this topic has focused on caffeine intake and delayed conception rather than long-term effects such as early menopause or age-related infertility. Very little has been done on the mechanism involved. Still the available evidence suggests women of reproductive age should limit their intake of caffeine.

For example, one study looked at caffeine consumption in five European countries and found those women who drank more than 500 milligrams of caffeine (roughly equivalent to five cups of coffee) per day had a much longer wait to get pregnant for the first time. Another smaller study showed women who consumed more than *one* cup of coffee per day (or caffeine equivalent) were half as likely to conceive during any given month than women who consumed less. Over a year's time, only 6 percent of women in the low consumption group had not conceived as compared with 28 percent in the high consumption group.

A study by the Harvard School of Public Health also showed an increase of risk of infertility due to tubal disease or endometriosis in women who consumed the caffeine equivalent of at least five cups of coffee per day. Finally, it's important to note that for women who are actively trying to conceive, and do so, limiting caffeine is imperative.

100

Here's why: moderate caffeine use (300 or more milligrams per day) has also been linked to premature and low birth weight infants; and just 151 or more milligrams per day is associated with an increased risk of miscarriage in the late first or second trimester of pregnancy.

Although I had limited understanding, I figured if effects could be seen with just one, two, or three cups of coffee, none would be even better for my chances to beat my clock. Unfortunately, I took this step a little too late. Still, I'm happy I'm no longer addicted to caffeine and constantly revved up on it. Though, I must admit, I still stop at Dunkin' Donuts to enjoy a frothy cappuccino—decaf, of course!

It appears that alcohol may have a similar, and possibly even a longer-term effect compared to caffeine. In one study, the results suggested caffeine might actually enhance alcohol's negative effect on conception. The message on alcohol is that it can delay conception and impact fertility. A recent report of more than 7,000 women in Sweden showed those who reported drinking a half a bottle of spirits, or a couple of bottles of wine per week, were at a substantial risk for seeing a fertility specialist as opposed to those who drank less. They also had a much lower number of first and second children than the others. The authors suggest, "It may be important for the female partner in an infertile couple to limit alcohol intake, or to not drink at all." Also, a Danish study of more than 400 women found that 64 percent of women who consumed less than one drink per day or less than five per week, conceived for the first time; but only 55 percent who drank more than six drinks per week achieved pregnancy.

At the moment, it is highly recommended that women trying to conceive restrict alcohol completely. If you are not actively trying to conceive, you'll probably be fine with low alcohol consumption, but it's important to understand that you may want to decrease or halt even social drinking as soon as you start thinking about trying to conceive. Yes, it would be a lot easier if they could make non-alcoholic beverages, especially wine, taste as good as decaf....

9. Reduce Stress

Life is full of stress. The quantity of it plus your ability to cope with it will determine how much of a role it plays in your health, including reproductive health. When I look back at my life when my son was conceived naturally, it was essentially stress-free and blissful. I had a

101

job I enjoyed, I was newly in love, and I was skiing in Vermont almost every weekend. Jump forward one year 10 months: I am married, a first time homeowner, and a new working mother. This period of time was anything but bliss. Given that my husband and I had little time together before we became parents, we had some rough times initially. No room for romance, some financial difficulties, and hardly any time to really get to know one another. The baby was the focus of our lives right out of the starting gates. Plus, I was now working two jobs (my own doing)—a full-time health reporting job during the week, plus covering everything from car crashes to snowstorms on weekends at a network affiliate in Boston. This amounted to a regular six- to seven-day workweek added to all the difficulties of scheduling daycare during odd hours, with my husband away weeks, sometimes a month at a time. But that's when I decided it was time to start trying for another baby. It didn't work.

Yes, my FSH tests revealed I had some serious "clock" issues, but when I think about the stress factor, it's extremely clear that the second time around was less than optimal for conception. Also, once I started trying, I was faced with impossible timing difficulties with my husband's work schedule that put him in the middle of the Gulf of Mexico when he should have been in bed with me. Plus the ultimate realization that my FSH was already in the hot zone, on top of the emotional and financial stress of failed treatment with frozen sperm to get around the timing issues, and it's no wonder we came up empty. Of course that *ticktock* never stopped, talk about stress!

Stress is a whole body phenomenon. It affects just about every working part, including the reproductive system. The body's reaction to stress is an output of hormones that turn on the "fight or flight" response and shuts down other areas such as the immune system and the reproductive system. In prehistoric times, this was a good thing. It allowed people to run fast and climb up trees to flee wild animals. Under chronically stressful conditions, this response also likely prevented reproduction or caused premature births, which meant there was no child to worry about.

Today this ancient hormonal response comes in handy in real emergency situations, when playing sports, or even when putting on your best presentation at the office. However, when things get rough at home or at the office, these days, we can't just run away. Though they might not be life threatening, we have to deal with many more stressors than our ancestors. And for some people they just keep piling on.

It is believed that when the body signals for an output of stress hormones, such as cortisol and adrenaline, they tell the hypothalamus to cut back on the reproductive hormones, GnRH (which triggers FSH), as well as progesterone. This throws the system off balance and can interfere with ovulation and menstruation. There are few studies that show a definitive link between stress and infertility, but there are dozens, if not hundreds, that highly suggest this relationship. The most recent evidence comes from the University of Pittsburgh School of Medicine, in women who have a condition called functional hypothalamic amenorrhea, or FHA. These are women who either have no menstrual cycles or have highly erratic periods, though they are of childbearing age and have no other medical condition related to infertility.

Researchers did blood tests on 22 women with FHA and 24 with normal menstrual cycles. They found all of the women with FHA had elevated levels of cortisol, a dangerous stress hormone, in their blood serum and in the fluid surrounding their brains and spinal cords. The cortisol concentrations in the cerebrospinal fluid were 30 percent higher in women with FHA than in those with normal periods. Blood serum cortisol levels were 23 percent higher.

Though FHA affects only about 5 percent of women of reproductive age, it illustrates a direct correlation between stress and its effect on the reproductive system. It is also important to point out that these women had no idea they were stressed out—even though cortisol was flowing through their bodies constantly. Sarah Berga, M.D., lead author of the study, says, "Typically these women are not aware they're under stress, or don't acknowledge it." The women described themselves as perfectionists, with high expectations of achievement.

The condition has now been shown to be associated with high stress-hormone levels, and can be reversed with stress reduction intervention. Experts point out that this is an extreme condition, and even though these women were unaware of their stress levels, their bodies showed undeniable consequences, that is, FHA. Some researchers speculate that stress, which is not high enough to cause amenorrhea, could interfere with fertility in more subtle ways even though women continue to menstruate.

Taking a look at the stress picture from the standpoint of infertility, the evidence is much more clear. No doubt about it, infertility *causes* stress, and all the hormonal responses that go along with it. So, if you are stressed out already, then decide you want to start trying for a baby, and are not successful immediately, guess what? More stress. If down the road you continue to be unsuccessful, then are faced with a slowing clock or other infertility diagnosis, stress can become a vicious cycle. Your stress hormones throw your entire system off balance, then you start compounding the problem with more stress due to the monthly baby-making emotional rollercoaster ride, and now you are in trouble.

Fortunately, though, it has been shown that people who are experiencing difficulty getting pregnant or going through infertility treatment can improve their chances through taking part in a support group. Back in 1990, researchers studied women who were the first to take part in a program aimed at reducing the stress of infertility. The program was based on teaching relaxation techniques that can be employed at any time during the day. The results of the first study showed that within six months of the program, 34 percent of the participants became pregnant. Nine years later, another similar, larger, study showed 42 percent of the women became pregnant within six months. Those who became pregnant tended to be younger and had more psychological distress when they entered the program. A longer-term project by the same researchers followed a group of infertile women and controls for a year. The results improved to 55 percent pregnant in those participating in the mind/body relaxation support group compared to just 20 percent in the control group.

This mind/body stress/infertility connection remains a mystery, but the available evidence gives you a basis for watching stress levels regardless of where you are in your reproductive planning. Too much stress is unhealthy. However, this is something you can generally control in a variety of ways: go for a bike ride, go skiing, jump in the ocean, sit down and imagine you are floating on a cloud, do something nice for someone, play with your dog or cat, go out to brunch with a good friend, etc. If you are experiencing a lot of stress in your life that you can't avoid, try a yoga class or join a support group.

About a year into my odyssey through the world of infertility, my home life and work life improved drastically. I joined a fabulous support group through RESOLVE, and as soon as I started my donor cycle, I also underwent acupuncture twice a week—this relaxed me more than the deepest sleep. I'll never know if it was a waste of time, but I'll also never know if it made an incredible difference.

10. Calculate Your Clock

If you don't read anything else in this book, read this, and do it. You won't find the following information anywhere else.

The first three calculations are critical and based on scientific evidence. The rest are founded on direct and indirect evidence and should be taken into account; the values presented can be used as guides.

First, you must determine how old your mother was when she went through menopause. If she hasn't gone through menopause, find out when your maternal grandmother (mother's mother) went through it. If neither age is available, you can look at the next closest maternal female relative. An aunt would do; an older sister would be better.

You can remind this person that menopause is the age she was when she had her last period, for good. The definition of menopause is *no period for a year*. So if she had one at 52, then had one six months later after she turned 53, then never had one again, the age at menopause is 53. Make sure you ask her to remember as precisely as possible, because this is very important. Here's why: Genetics are the best predictor of when you will go through menopause. Research has shown that 80 percent of the time, a daughter will go through menopause at the same age as her mother. Studies of twins also corroborate this, because identical twins go through the menopause at the same age. So knowing your mother's age at menopause gives you an 80 percent likelihood of going through menopause at the same time, and you can then estimate when you will also experience dropping off the fertility cliff. Your mother probably didn't care about the cliff part because she likely had her children long before that happened. She probably has no idea when she lost her fertility, she thinks it happened the last time she had her period, and she would be about *10 years* off the mark.

That's right, on average, a woman's fertility takes a steep decline at about 10 years prior to her very last period. If you think of it in terms of a clock, this is when the clock stops keeping time; and like a clock, the hands might move from time to time, so yes, it is still possible to get pregnant, but the clock is junk, it's not to be depended upon at this point. Physiologically, on average, this is also the time when FSH levels begin to steadily rise, and egg quality steadily declines—even though you may have regular periods.

If you can get an accurate answer from your mother or other female relative, then you have taken a major step toward calculating the true life span of your biological clock. If your mother's age at menopause was 51, which is the average, for all intents and purposes, she probably lost her fertility at age 41, which is what you can count on as a base. If your mother went through menopause later, at, say, age 55, you could be one of the lucky ones who might have a little extra time in your early 40s. Also, if your mother smoked, estimate that her age at menopause should have been two to three years later, so subtract 10 years from that age.

Of course, there is the other 20 percent of cases that don't follow the same genetic pattern as their mothers, so statistically if you fall into that category, you could be older or younger than this estimate when your fertility drops. However, the odds are that you will be very close.

Starting at the average base of age 41 for your fertility decline, you can then begin subtracting time for the rust you might have accumulated—that is, damage or other insults your clock may have endured over the years. The most important one is smoking. This is the next best predictor of fertility loss. If you've smoked for any length of time, or are currently smoking, subtract another two to three years. (Research shows it can be anywhere from one to four years). So, be somewhat conservative and take away three years; now you are down to age 38. This is your best estimate for the absolute deadline for having your family. If you haven't had all the children you want by the time you are 38, you may run into difficulty, especially if you keep smoking.

The research on quitting has been mixed, some studies suggest quitting will bring back the ability to get pregnant into normal ranges, others indicate that smoking can do permanent damage. After carefully reviewing this literature, however, it's clear that smoking destroys eggs, and the fewer eggs you have, the quicker you may lose your fertility. So if you have smoked and quit, you might want to subtract a year or two, to be on the safe side.

There are a few more important smoking variables that you should throw into this equation. They are: (1) secondhand smoke, and (2) whether your mother smoked when she was pregnant with you. The data in this area is less precise, especially concerning sec-ondhand smoke. Again, knowing how susceptible the ovaries are to toxins in cigarette smoke, it makes sense that if you are constantly exposed to someone else's smoke, there is a potential risk to your eggs.

Also, though there's no research, it's important to point out that many adults have been exposed to their parents' secondhand smoke as children. I was one of them. My house was constantly filled with smoke, as was the car, and many of my parents' friends' homes. It was everywhere, and there was no escape. This may not do as much dam-age as your own smoking, but it is something you should be aware of. If you have all the eggs you are ever going to get at birth (or all the ovarian stem cells that produce eggs, as new research suggests), pas-sive smoking at any age has the potential to chip away at that precious resource. Jonathan Tilly, mentioned earlier, agrees, "Maybe it would take longer for that person breathing secondhand smoke to be af-fected than somebody directly inhaling the tobacco smoke, but none-theless, the chemicals are there and they're not a good thing."

If you have ever been subjected to constant exposure to second-hand smoke, whether currently or in the distant past, it may be pru-dent to take another six months off your clock. Now we are down to age 37.5.

Next, you have to ask your mother what could be a very conten-tious question. Try to ease into it so you can get an honest answer. In a very nonconfrontational way ask her, "Mom, just curious, did you ever smoke when you were pregnant with me?"

Before I get to why this is so important, I want to tell you that for a very long time, I spent a considerable amount of time wondering "why?" Why did I have a baby at 40, a perfectly healthy baby, after an impeccable pregnancy, and one year later, I couldn't have another? I knew there had to be a reasonable answer; I couldn't accept "unex-plained" infertility. I just had a baby! One night, wide-awake and los-ing sleep over my newly discovered infertility, I remembered my doctor asking me if I had ever smoked. Of course I answered emphatically, "NO, NEVER." In fact, I absolutely hated smoking, perhaps because I could never get away from it as a child. Then all of a sudden, a lightbulb went on! Visions of our smoke-filled kitchen, my father's cigars, my mother's cigarettes, flashed through my mind. I came back to the present for a moment and said to myself, "Hmmmm, if smoking can corrode the biological clock, all that passive smoke as a child might have an impact, but hey wait a minute—my eggs formed when I was developing inside my mother—as she was lighting up cigarette after cigarette." Logically, I thought, if the smoke could have damaged her eggs, could it have damaged mine *even before I was born*?" The answer, I now trust, is yes.

Remember cotinine? It has been found in the hair of babies directly following their birth. Researchers in France studied hair samples from 182 mothers and their newborns (they had to exclude 50 other newborns because they didn't have enough hair to test!). Nicotine and cotinine concentrations were measured at birth. In the mothers, both nicotine and cotinine concentrations were associated with cigarette smoking during the last trimester. In their newborns, cotinine levels were also associated with the number of cigarettes their mothers smoked during the third trimester. If it gets in the babies' hair, it's managed to go everywhere else too.

Obviously, it's difficult to look at the ovaries of these newborns to see any effects, and it would be even more impossible to study ovaries of fetuses before they are born. Not so in mice. Thanks to these little creatures, it is possible get a better idea of what could be happening to our eggs as we develop and our mothers are smoking.

The same Massachusetts General Hospital team that showed PAHs (polycyclic aromatic hydrocarbons), a toxin found in high concentrations in cigarette smoke, can kill human eggs also looked at how the toxin affects the ovaries of female *fetal* mice. They found that even a slight exposure of the fetuses to PAHs in utero (while still in their mothers' bodies) resulted in baby girl mice with *substantially fewer eggs* than those not exposed. Two other studies have also come to the same conclusion. The finding is significant especially given that the dose of PAHs needed to trigger extensive egg death in the fetal ovaries is far less than the amount of the chemical required to cause similar amounts of egg death following birth.

This could spell tremendous trouble for women exposed to their mother's smoke in utero. The authors say, "Even a brief window of exposure of the fetal ovaries to PAHs, such as that which probably occurs when women smoke while pregnant, would be sufficient to cause irreparable long-term harm to the developing germ line." Tilly points to other important work that looked at PAH exposure during different ages in the female mouse. "In utero exposure was the worst developmental window—we needed very little of this stuff to essentially wipe out all the fetal egg cells. That amount of chemical does nothing in adults."

Just a couple more points about this. If your mother smoked and you were breast-fed, you were also likely exposed to tobacco toxins through breast milk as well. Cotinine has been found in breast milk, and also in the urine of babies who were breast-fed by their mothers. The concentrations depended on the number of cigarettes smoked—with the highest concentrations in the urine of babies who were fully breast-fed. So much for all that healthful breast milk!

It has been known for years that smoking while pregnant causes a higher incidence of low birth-weight babies and babies born small for gestational age. It turns out that new research is finding that teenage girls who were smaller at birth have a tendency not to ovulate. One study shows a substantial number of girls who were small at birth did not ovulate at all, even though they had their period for at least the previous three years; and those that did ovulate, did so much slower than normal controls. Other work has shown that women who were lighter at birth have smaller ovaries—that is, fewer eggs—and are less sensitive to follicle-stimulating hormone.

The last bit of information to share is the evidence that many of the women who are having the most difficulty trying to get pregnant had been exposed to tobacco smoke long, long ago. A few studies show a significantly reduced ability to conceive in women who reported being exposed to tobacco smoke in utero. These studies come to the same conclusion: women whose mothers smoked while pregnant with them may have much more difficulty getting and staying pregnant than women whose mothers did not smoke during pregnancy.

If your mother smoked while pregnant with you, take another two to three years off your clock. This is just a guess, but if it's up to four years if you smoke, and it likely takes less toxin to affect a fetus's eggs than an adult's, then two years is probably a reasonable, if not low, estimate. Now you are down to 35.5.

Any major exposure that you know of to other environmental toxins, you may want to take another six months off. Bringing you to age 35.

Finally, you should get a little time for good behavior. If you eat a fabulous daily diet full of antioxidants, actively reduce stress, avoid caffeine, and keep alcohol to a minimum, add a year. So there you are: age 36 is your deadline.

Now, of course, none of this will matter a bit if you decide to have children in your 20s, particularly early to mid-20s. You can smoke (although there are lots of other reasons not to) and probably not have any trouble, because you will likely have enough good eggs to make it to 30, perhaps a couple years beyond that. But if you are college educated, planning on a career, then marriage for a few years, then children sometime in your 30s, use this as a guide, and plan your future family so that you don't face this heart-wrenching, stress-producing, tear-inducing, earlier than expected, unforgiving, time-bomb of a biological clock.

Review: How to Calculate Your Clock

_____1. Get accurate age of how old your mother was at menopause (remember to add two to three years if she smoked).

_____2. Subtract 10 years for approximate age your clock will stop, or you will encounter extremely unreliable fertility.

_____3. Subtract two to three years if you are/were a smoker.

_____4. Subtract six months for lots of secondhand smoke exposure.

_____5. Subtract another two to three years for fetal exposure to tobacco smoke.

_____6. Subtract six months for known toxin exposures.

_____7. Add one year for healthy lifestyle (great diet, low stress, low or no caffeine, or alcohol).

_____
Target age to complete your family.

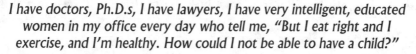

THE "ARTs"

5.

I have doctors, Ph.D.s, I have lawyers, I have very intelligent, educated women in my office every day who tell me, "But I eat right and I exercise, and I'm healthy. How could I not be able to have a child?"

—Dr. Marcelle Cedars to Lesley Stahl on *60 Minutes,* June 2002

The Age of ART

Assisted reproductive technology (ART) has made tremendous strides since the first IVF baby was born more than two decades ago. Indeed, ART has helped countless couples realize their dream of having a family—including those struggling with their naturally plummeting fertility. But generally, those who defy the clock are the lottery winners, the fortunate few. Within the world of reproductive medicine, conquering age-related infertility is the Holy Grail, the mission driving researchers to their laboratory benches each day. It is the final frontier of reproductive science, because at the moment, there's only so much medicine can do.

If you have high FSH, have reached age 35, or are simply curious, this chapter will provide a no-nonsense look at fertility treatment aimed at a very specific group of women: those over age 35 or those whose clocks are approaching the fertility equivalent of Cinderella's midnight hour. If this is you, it doesn't matter how well you eat, how often you exercise, or how young you look, you will more than likely have less time, fewer options, and a more difficult road to travel to reach your goal of creating a family.

You may have heard about celebrities, possibly friends, or even family members who have gone through fertility treatment, but you probably never learned the whole story. It is a delicate subject that few enjoy talking about, and not many are bold enough to ask about. This is your opportunity to walk through the doors of the ART world, look around, and assess for yourself whether you should run to your awaiting horse-drawn chariot well before the stroke of midnight rather than push it and find you're suddenly left with a pumpkin and useless mice, and no alternative but to embark on a long walk down an uncertain and painfully rocky road to achieve your dreams of having a child.

A Typical Success Story

Abby and John had been together for several years, including three years of marriage. Both are physicians in top Harvard affiliated teaching hospitals in Boston. Like so many well-educated couples, they waited to establish their careers before having a family.

After a solid year of trying on their own, they sought help. Diagnostic testing quickly showed Abby was having difficulty due to age. She couldn't believe it; they both thought they planned their lives perfectly. Even with their dozen years of medical training combined, they were mistaken. They had no idea they could have such trouble starting a family—after all, they were in the prime of their lives, both in their mid-30s.

I met Abby when I was admitted to a Boston hospital with kidney stones in the middle of writing Chapter 2—I was 24 weeks pregnant. She just happened to be in the same hospital room and was 35 weeks along. She told me her story.

She had been through several IVF cycles before she became pregnant with twins. The pregnancy marched along perfectly, but at 27 weeks she went into early labor. Doctors alleviated her labor, but they confined her to total bed rest. This meant leaving her job—indefinitely.

Eventually she developed gestational diabetes, high blood pressure, and preeclampsia. That night she faced danger. The doctors knew it; she knew it. If the babies stayed put, her health could be in jeopardy, and if they were born, the babies could face lifelong medical problems. This bright, successful, young woman had worked diligently to have these children, and now at this late stage, they were putting her health at risk.

That evening, I heard her crying. My heart sank. I thought, *How heart wrenching—this woman is just* 36 *years old, near the end of her pregnancy with babies she wanted so much, she endured cycle after cycle of fertility treatment. And she was lucky. She got pregnant with her own eggs.*

Holding back the tears, she told me to make sure younger women know that even if they are successful with technology in their 30s, it's not necessarily all roses. The infertility treatment merry-go-round is difficult on the career, the relationship, and life in general. Even when you are blessed with a pregnancy, there's always a good chance for a bonus—*multiples*—which carries greater risk for complications. If she and her husband had understood the biological clock, Abby may have taken an FSH test, they may have embarked on their family sooner, and avoided this difficult situation.

Taking Action With Assistance if Your Clock Is Nearly Stopped

Fast-forward two more years, and Abby may not have been as fortunate. Had this couple waited even longer, or delayed entering treatment, Abby might have missed *her* chance to have her own genetic children. It happens all the time. When the clock begins to wind down, there is no time to waste. As soon as you suspect a problem, even if your OB-GYN tells you to keep trying, insist on an FSH test, and if you get a borderline result, head straight to a reputable reproductive medicine clinic for treatment. (Remember, your husband can have his own genetic children well into his golden years. But you will lose that luxury—it can happen suddenly and sometimes at a surprisingly young age.)

Single women too. Whether you are in a relationship or not, if you have borderline FSH, or are over 35, you may want to ask yourself this question: if having my own genetic child is now or never, would I prefer *never*? One of the largest clinics in the Boston area has a steady flow of single professional women passing through its doors simply to survey their options. Having a child while you are fertile with simple IUI (intrauterine insemination, also known as artificial insemination) using donated sperm is much easier than waiting and having to go through IVF, or even thinking about using both donated eggs *and* sperm.

If you decide single motherhood is not for you, at least you will be able to make your decision based on solid information. You might conclude that genetics are not that important, and if you eventually meet Mr. Right, you would consider a family with him through the use of donor eggs, or adoption. Either way, do what's right for you knowing that your clock will do what it's destined to, no matter what you choose or when.

Shot, Shots, and More Shots

I'll never forget the first visit to my reproductive endocrinologist following my FSH test. At the time, I had no idea what the results meant. I just knew it wasn't very good news. He said to me, "We can start with a couple of stimulated IUIs and see what happens."

I said, "Okay, what does that mean, *stimulated*?"

He said, "Well, we'll give you some fertility medications you inject twice a day...."

I stopped him, "What? Inject? You mean I have to give myself a shot?"

"Yes. Don't you want to do it?" he replied.

"Well, sure, but isn't there a pill I can take?" I asked.

He paused and looked at me, and in a friendly, but concerned tone, said, "Cara, you are waaaaay past pills."

Okay, so there I was a few weeks later, at about 9 o'clock at night with all the medications prepared, ready to give myself the first shot. Generally, husbands are there to make this first injection a bit easier, but alas, mine was at work on his ship. So no help from him! Although, I think I called him about 10 times that night.

Needle in hand, pointed at my thigh, ready to jab—and nothing. I tried again, and couldn't do it. Over the phone my husband kept saying,

114

"Just do it! Just do it!" Call me a coward, but I couldn't *just do it*. I started to panic, because these shots had to be taken at around the same time each morning and night. Finally, I gave up. I woke up my 18-month-old son, grabbed the needle and medications, jumped in the car, and rushed to my mother's house 40 minutes away. By that time it was 10:30—and the drug had probably lost some of its effectiveness—but I needed help. Luckily she was up, and had no trouble sticking me in the thigh. We laughed, and recalled the time she promised to pierce my ears, but nearly fainted after the first ear. Anyway, I stayed overnight, so she could do the morning shot too. Finally, the next night, I was able to stick myself.

If you never had the experience of injecting yourself, you may have difficulty the first or second time. However, I can assure you, it gets much easier. I learned later that a bit of ice on the injection spot for a minute beforehand eliminates any sensation from the needle. I promise, eventually you don't even need that. In fact, the shots become the simplest step, precisely mixing the drug and removing it from the tiny ampoule is the nerve-wracking part of the procedure.

Age and "Take-Home-Baby" Rates

Most women who either haven't come across someone who has had difficulties achieving pregnancy, or have somehow been misinformed about their biological clocks, believe that reproductive medicine clinics can make miracles happen—all the time. The fact is, in younger women—that is, women under 40—more times than not, treatment still fails. On average, *60* out of 100 women fail to get pregnant, even with the best technology, and under the best conditions. This is hardly perfect science.

The graph on page 116 illustrates the CDC's 2001 statistics (every year this graph looks essentially the same), showing just how sharp the decline in live birth rates is, starting in the late 20s, dropping throughout the late 30s and early 40s *with* reproductive technology.

Each year the CDC reports national averages for live births per cycle of treatment, in addition to other related reproductive outcomes. In 2001, for women under age 35, the proportion of cycles resulting in a live baby was just 35 percent; for women ages 35 to 37, only 28 percent took home babies; for women 38 to 40, just under 20 percent fulfilled their dreams of parenthood; and only 10.4 percent of women ages 41 to 42 walked out of the hospital with a newborn. Substantially more women in the last category got pregnant, but nearly half of them miscarried.

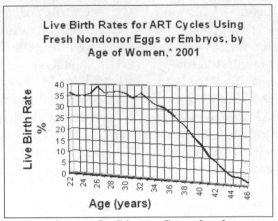

Of course, these are national averages, statistics based on more than 77,000 cycles using fresh embryos from non-donor eggs. The data illustrate an important point

Source: Centers for Disease Control and Prevention Website (*www.cdc.gov/reproductive health/ART01/sect2*).

about age. The younger you are, the better your chances for a child. As one top reproductive endocrinologist put it, "We think that technologically can control many things about our lives, and this translates into reproductive biology and reproductive health. But that is not necessarily the case. At the end of the day, people need to understand, the earlier one tries to achieve a pregnancy, the better off one is."

So before reading any further, think *age*. Much of what technology can do is dependent on it. After 35 there is generally time for one baby/pregnancy, but maybe not two. After 40, in general, you are very fortunate to have one; it's rare to have two. However, the sooner you enlist a specialist, the faster you will be able to learn how efficiently your particular clock is running.

Getting Started

There are really only two ways to know if you should seek out a reproductive endocrinologist. The more traditional way is coming up empty after having unprotected (preferably timed) intercourse for a year, or the less traditional way, getting your FSH and E2 tested even before you start trying. The standard year of trying "the old-fashioned way" is appropriate for women under 35; however, OB-GYNs and reproductive endocrinologists alike, recommend if you are 35 or over, six months is enough time to try on your own without success. Some OB-GYNs give 40-plus women the same advice. While you may get lucky and become pregnant, if I were 40, or even in my late 30s, knowing what I know now, I'd go to a clinic and have some diagnostic testing done *while* trying. Even six months can make a difference when you've reached your late 30s or early 40s. Besides, it takes at least a month to get an appointment, and then it's generally another month or two before your cycle rolls around to do your blood tests on the third day of your period.

Infertility Specialist or Board Certified Reproductive Endocrinologist?

If you are under age 35 and your OB-GYN treats infertility, you may feel comfortable remaining in his or her care; however, if your FSH is in the borderline range, or if you are older, you may be better off moving on to a clinic and seeing an RE. These women wish they had:

After I got married at 40, we tried to conceive for a year, and my OB-GYN simply said we were doing it wrong. She never even tested me to find out if I was ovulating. I finally went to an RE, and was told, "Your eggs are too old. You will need an egg donor. Here's a list of agencies."

— Jennifer, age 41

I started skipping periods in my early 30s. Two different OB-GYNs dismissed my concerns saying it was just stress. I'm now 38, have had seven treatment cycles, two of them miscarried, the rest were cancelled or failed. Now two REs have said my problems started with those missed periods. I'm devastated.

—Carol, age 38

Here are the major differences between an obstetrician-gynecologist who treats infertility and an RE. After graduating from medical school, it takes a four-year residency to become an OB-GYN. The amount of time these residents spend in fertility training ranges from eight to 12 weeks. However, if an OB-GYN goes into reproductive endocrinology and wants to become board certified, that means another three years in a fellowship, and at least 18 to 24 months in hands-on clinical training. So the disparity is three months of fertility training versus 27 months. To become an RE, a candidate also has to go through two rounds of written and oral exams to become board certified in obstetrics and gynecology as well as reproductive endocrinology. You can decide which you would rather entrust the creation of your family to when you may be running out of time.

That doesn't mean to say that OB-GYNs can't help. Often they can, but you want to make sure they understand the age-related fertility decline. If you are considering remaining with a trusted OB-GYN, he or she may be more knowledgeable and willing to make referrals sooner if affiliated with a reproductive medicine clinic.

Choosing a Reproductive Medicine Clinic and an RE

This is probably one of the most important early decisions you will make; it is also the most difficult. If there is little choice, go to the clinic that is within your reach. Don't assume that you must live in a major metropolitan city to have access to the best programs. There are good clinics across the country.

The best method for finding the clinics near you is the CDC Website (see Resources) and search in your home state or nearby states. It is important you choose a clinic that is relatively convenient, or make arrangements to stay near the clinic you decide upon. You will be making many trips for doctor's appointments and diagnostic tests; and during your treatment cycle(s), several visits for monitoring; and for your IUI or egg retrieval; and later for embryo transfer.

In addition to clinic locations, the CDC Website also provides individual program statistics. You may want to look over the statistics; however, if you are age 35 or over, try to resist making your decision based on success rates alone. Many clinics will have lower success rates simply because they *will* treat older women with higher FSH levels. These clinics take on borderline cases; their doctors put the couples' wishes ahead of their success rates. So sometimes the best clinic for someone over 35 with an elevated FSH is not the one with the highest success rate, it is the clinic that will be most aggressive treating *you*.

Many clinics err on the side of caution and will discourage treatment, especially if you are age 40 or over and have an elevated FSH, or fail a Clomid Challenge Test. Some will outright refuse to treat you using your own eggs. Success rates are usually the priority in these clinics. It doesn't matter whether you can afford several treatment cycles for your slim chance at parenthood; in states where infertility is covered by insurance, the clinic still won't risk lowering its success rates for your opportunity to create your own genetic child.

Often the chances in borderline cases can be 5 percent or less. Be sure you know where a clinic stands before you waste your time and go through extensive, expensive diagnostic testing, only to be told they can't help you, and you must locate another clinic and do it all over again. Try to find a clinic and doctor who will test you, provide accurate information on the results along with possible success rates given your age and—this is really important—allow *you* to make the decision whether to move forward with treatment.

Dr. Zev Rosenwaks, director of the Center for Reproductive Medicine and Infertility at the Weill Medical College at Cornell University, says many women who can get pregnant never have the opportunity because clinics won't take the chance. He insists, "If somebody has an FSH in the menopausal range, then they shouldn't do IVF. But if they have a borderline FSH, they don't have a zero chance ever. The same goes for someone who fails the Clomid Challenge Test. She doesn't have a zero chance." Rosenwaks points to a woman who was in her early 30s who had an FSH of 70, and was diagnosed with premature menopause. "She was taking hormonal medications to prepare for a treatment cycle using donor eggs, she ovulated, and got pregnant on her own, despite such a high FSH level," he says.

There are clinics, such as Rosenwaks's, that take borderline cases, and also have high success rates. Unfortunately, unless you have unlimited financial resources, and are willing to travel, you may not be able to access such a clinic. The next best thing is to locate the clinics that are a possibility for you, then scour the data for your age category. Those treating the most women in your age category, and reporting the highest success rates, are the best bets. Some clinics will also have more current success rate data than the CDC, so be sure to ask for it.

One more thing: some clinics will do extensive treatment when the chances are extremely remote. Any clinic that is eager to do IVF when your FSH and other diagnostic tests strongly indicate less than a 10 percent chance of success (often odds are less than 5 percent) may not be looking out for your best interests. When you are paying out of pocket, it is important to make sure you weigh your potential success rate objectively, and allocate your financial resources carefully, so you will be able to at least consider donor eggs or adoption, if treatment with your own eggs fails. Most reputable clinics will discuss this with you, usually with a financial expert and an experienced psychologist or social worker to help you with these difficult decisions.

Now, to find a doctor within a clinic, the first rule is to resist going to the RE who has the earliest appointment. Even though it feels critical to start immediately, it is better to find the *right* doctor than to book quickly with the *wrong* doctor. Call the clinics for information. Ask about all their doctors: Who takes the most women over 35? Who is most aggressive with borderline cases?

The second rule for finding a doctor in your situation is to remember you need *cutting-edge*, not Dr. John Smith, who uses the same basic protocol on every patient. Therefore, don't be surprised if the top-notch RE you want to see is booked for a month or two. Make the appointment. Be patient, many REs report upwards of 50 percent of their patients are women 35 and over; it's no surprise the best doctors for such cases are in high demand.

Another good way to learn about the clinics, their philosophies, and individual doctors, is by contacting members of your local chapter of Resolve: The National Infertility Association. If the notion of an *infertility* advocacy group makes you nervous, try to get over it. This organization is a great resource for anyone who has any kind of question about *fertility*, and the local clinics that deal with it. There are always volunteers willing to talk. If you don't get someone on the phone immediately, keep trying and leave a message. In my experience, they always get back to you.

The "35 and Over" Infertility Workup

In addition to documenting your health history and your reproductive history, your RE will want to run a battery of tests to determine if there is any hint of diminished ovarian reserve—that is, a slowing clock—or any other problem that might interfere with conception. The tests will include many you learned about in Chapter 1, plus others. These tests are tremendously valuable to help your RE establish a potential treatment plan for you.

120

Currently there are great discrepancies in the literature and among top REs as to which combinations of these tests are most worthwhile. Some recent studies claim that while the standard FSH and E2 tests are valuable, performing a vaginal ultrasound and counting the antral follicles best indicates how effectively your ovaries will respond to treatment. Other research has come to the conclusion that the standard tests along with an additional Clomid Challenge Test provide the most optimal look at your clock. Still many swear by the inhibin B test as the "tie-breaker" when results of the FSH and E2 tests are inconclusive. One reputable RE says unless the case is extremely complicated, all you need is the FSH/E2 combination along with age of the woman to determine how best to proceed with ART, adding that the rest of the tests are a waste of time and money. However, if you were to have each test done, the results would become part of a biological clock puzzle. How the pieces fit together gives you and your RE a clearer picture of where you are on the clock dial. The closer you are to Cinderella's midnight, the more aggressive your treatment should be.

Timing Is Critical

These tests are important to establish the best course in treatment, because you don't want to waste time with ineffective procedures. Still, all initial diagnostic tests should be performed over one or two months at the most. If you are 35 or over, your RE should put you on the diagnostic fast track to starting the most appropriate treatment as quickly as possible.

Ready, Set, Go!

Think of assisted reproduction treatment options as rungs of a ladder. The lowest rungs are the "pills" I referred to earlier. Popping prescription Clomid to tap on your ovaries and politely ask them to produce a good egg or two, while timing intercourse to coincide with ovulation, is lightweight treatment, even if you enlist an RE to monitor your cycle with hormone tests and ultrasounds. If you are over 35 and are having difficulty, this may not be your best option. Still, depending on how borderline your fertility is, and your available financial resources, you may opt to start on this first rung. Prescription

In women age 40 or over with high FSH, the picture is relatively bleak, though not entirely hopeless. In one study, of 93 patients who were either 41 or older, and/or had an elevated FSH, 88 began treatment for IVF. Only five with an FSH of 15 or greater made it to egg retrieval. Doctors gathered an average of only three eggs from each woman. Unfortunately, none conceived. Another study looked at a group of confirmed poor responders who had already failed a previous IVF cycle. These 63 women underwent a subsequent stimulation cycle using a different protocol. This time, they produced more eggs, resulting in many more embryos to choose from and transfer— ultimately, seven viable pregnancies resulted.

In fact, many women have conceived with elevated FSH. Although the chances are remote, some hit the jackpot. Any professional in the reproduction field can relate cases of women who conceived when the odds dictated it was next to impossible. In low probability situations, couples and their doctors must carefully assess the treatment options, the stress they induce, the odds of success, and the costs of exercising their choices, before proceeding.

Basic Treatment Options for Older Patients and Poor Responders

Once it is determined that your fertility is at least somewhat impaired and you are a candidate for stimulation with injectable fertility medications, you will decide whether to try the drug protocols with intrauterine insemination (IUI), or go straight to IVF. Many REs will offer stimulation with IUI for one to three cycles if your FSH is not more than 12, and other tests show probability of good response, so long as you are no older than 38. However, even in this borderline but relatively hopeful case, many REs will suggest moving straight into IVF. Starting with IUI can be more attractive though, given the lower cost, when the chances for success are in the 20- to 30-percent range. Generally, a stimulated IUI cycle including medications can run $1500 to $3500, whereas you can expect to spend three to four times that for each IVF cycle.

One drawback to stimulated IUI is the inability to limit the number of eggs that will be ovulated. If you stimulate well, and several follicles mature, they will all be ovulated at the same time. The inseminations will take place usually over two days following ovulation, and therefore sperm may fertilize more than one egg, possibly producing a multiple gestation. Generally, however, in women whose ovarian reserve is in decline, this is not a great concern. Rather, the more eggs the better, and if one produces a pregnancy, it is considered a tremendous success.

If you are nearing 40 or over, and desire a child, start trying on your own immediately, but more than likely, you should get to a reproductive medicine clinic for evaluation. At this age, there is typically little time to waste, regardless of what you've been led to believe by how fit you are for your biological age, or your general health. It is your clock, your reproductive *ovarian* age that counts. My doctor once said, "Look at you, you look great for 41, but your eggs are like little old ladies walking around with canes!" Also, don't be swayed by others who have had babies well into their 40s, even if they grace the covers of magazines. (More on this in Chapter 6.) Generally, you don't know if they hit the mega-million dollar lottery, how much they struggled to succeed, or if they simply used donor eggs. Think about *your* clock, and remember, it will slow to a crawl without fanfare, and can stop in terms of fertility without any warning.

What Is Ovarian Stimulation and Monitoring?

The stimulation portion of the treatment (referred to as controlled ovarian hyperstimulation, or COH) involves the injection of one or more kinds of FSH medication. You will likely be instructed to inject the medication twice a day for several days. These two shots will be spaced so that you have one at about the same time in the morning, and at night to keep the level of hormone in your system relatively constant.

Some forms of this medication are already premixed in liquid form. You carefully draw the exact dose out of a small bottle, and then inject it. More often, FSH comes in tiny doses of 75 IU (international units) in powdered form contained in separate small glass ampoules; these you snap open and mix yourself. Older women or those with predicted poor response will require two or three ampoules per shot. The maximum recommended dose is 450 IU per day, or six ampoules.

Learning to break open the little glass containers and mix the medications using a syringe and saline solution is cumbersome at first.

It is like having a science experiment to complete each morning and evening. Also, considering each daily dose can amount to hundreds of dollars, the pressure mounts with each plunge of the syringe.

Most women follow this two shot per day regimen for about four to eight days, sometimes more, during which your RE will begin daily monitoring of your response. On monitoring days, you will have an estrogen blood test and a vaginal ultrasound. Expect to feel poked and prodded more than ever during monitoring. Each day you will endure two or three shots, plus another needle prick for the blood test, and have an ultrasound probe inserted into your vagina to check on your follicles.

Just remember, careful monitoring is *essential* during stimulated cycles. One RE compared it to grilling a steak, "You have to constantly check on it, otherwise you run the risk of overcooking it, and that would be disastrous!" Come to think of it, given how poked and prodded you feel, the steak analogy is right on target!

Kidding aside, the blood estrogen levels will tell your RE how ready your follicles are for ovulation, and the ultrasound will allow her to measure their size. Once E2 levels reach an appropriate level and your follicles are large enough, you will be instructed to stop all shots and inject yourself with another drug called hCG (human chorionic gonadotropin) to coax your eggs into completing their maturation for IVF, or also induce ovulation for IUI. Monitoring is extremely time-intensive. Usually appointments are scheduled early in the morning, for at least two or three, but up to several consecutive days.

Suppression During Stimulation

Either prior to, or following the start of, your follicle-stimulating medications, your RE will also prescribe another injectable medication that will suppress a hormone called luteinizing hormone, or LH. These medications are called gonadotropin-releasing hormone agonists (GnRH agonist) or gonadotropin-releasing hormone antagonists (GnRH antagonist). These drugs are also injected subcutaneously, and depending on which protocol your doctor recommends, you may be giving yourself this shot once a day for several days leading up to the start of your stimulating medications, and for several days in conjunction with them. Other protocols require fewer injections.

126

Each type of medication works on LH via a different mechanism, but the result is that LH along with natural FSH is prevented from being released from the pituitary gland. This allows the injected FSH to push the ovaries to produce follicles to the maximum extent possible. When a GnRH agonist drug is begun prior to a stimulated cycle, it essentially provides a hormonal "clean slate" for the injected FSH to work with. In other protocols, the aim is simply to prevent the natural LH surge, which causes ovulation, so that more eggs are allowed to mature prior to IUI or egg retrieval for IVF. Without this drug-induced LH suppression, the stimulated eggs might naturally ovulate, and your RE would be unable to time your IUI, or prior to IVF, some or all of the eggs would be lost, egg retrieval would be impossible, and your cycle would be canceled.

There are many types of treatment protocols utilizing myriad drugs; the most basic protocols involve three types of medications: (1) those that *suppress* certain hormones, (2) those that *stimulate* follicles, and (3) hCG to *trigger* final maturation of the follicles. The standard treatment options vary in terms of the type, the start day, and the duration of the *suppression* medications. Among the various protocols, the stimulation portion of the treatment (FSH medication) remains fairly constant once your RE determines the amount you will need to produce the greatest number of mature eggs.

Exactly how these GnRH agonists or antagonists and FSH medications are prescribed varies from doctor to doctor and patient to patient. A good RE, who is up-to-date with the ever-changing research in this field, will be more apt to recommend more cutting-edge protocols for older women or predicted poor responders. The next several sections will give you an overview of the protocols that *seem* to be most effective for those experiencing an age-related decline in fertility. It is important to note that few REs will agree on which protocol is the *best* for poor responders. That's because the research is still evolving, and the precise definition of "poor responder" has yet to be decided.

The GnRH "Antagonist" Protocol

The GnRH antagonist drugs are the most recent main ingredients added to the RE's cupboard of recipe choices. The most commonly prescribed GnRH antagonist, Antagon, became available in the United

States in 2000. A few years later, research has begun to show treatment using a GnRH antagonist in conjunction with FSH-stimulating medications is likely the better option for patients who have either failed other treatments, are deemed potentially poor responders, or are dealing with advanced maternal age. (The technical term for "older patient" is advanced maternal age, or AMA, and some clinics call AMA 38-plus, others apply the distinction to those 40-plus.)

In the GnRH antagonist protocol, the FSH medication, usually at the highest dose of 450 IU, is started during the early part of the menstrual cycle, typically on the second or third day. (The first day of actual bleeding represents the beginning of the new cycle, even though the blood is the fallout from the previous cycle.) The GnRH antagonist is then begun on or about the 6th day of your stimulation with FSH; that's approximately when your monitoring usually reveals your dominant or largest follicle has reached about 14 millimeters in diameter. The GnRH antagonist will prevent the natural LH surge that can bring on maturation and ovulation, so that the dominant follicle, as well as the other smaller follicles, can continue growing without ovulating too soon. When enough follicles reach 18 to 20 millimeters, you will be directed to stop all medications and deliver the hCG shot to trigger final maturation and ovulation. Your IUI will take place over the next two days, or your eggs will be retrieved within exactly 34 to 36 hours for IVF.

This protocol differs substantially from the more standard treatments that have been in use for many years and have been very effective in patients that are normal responders. One major difference: using the antagonist protocol reduces the number of injections by 80 percent, according to one study. Not only that, new research is showing this option is more effective in poor responders for reasons that are not well understood. Researchers believe the GnRH antagonists permit nature to assist in the recruitment of your follicles. Because they are given later in the cycle, antagonists allow the body's early *natural* FSH to rise, to help kick-start the follicles' growth while still effectively suppressing the LH as the follicles continue their development. Mounting data shows that poor responders who have failed previous cycles on *agonist* protocols will produce more follicles on *antagonist* protocols.

One recent study involving poor responders shows the viable pregnancy rate per embryo transfer was nearly 24 percent in a group

128

undergoing treatment with GnRH antagonists, compared to just 7 percent in a group using GnRH agonists in their stimulation protocols. This is one of the more dramatic comparisons. There have been others showing antagonists are slightly better or at least equally as effective as some agonist protocols. Keep in mind these studies are few, and generally small, so have relative merit. As more research comparing protocols is published, eventually one method that is most beneficial for older, more challenging patients is expected to emerge.

The Agonist "Flare" Protocols

Prior to the availability of antagonists, many REs favored what's called a "flare" protocol in poor responders. This method of stimulation involves beginning agonist injections on the second day of the cycle to cause a sudden discharge, or "flare," of FSH and LH in the body. The FSH medication is started the next day. The idea is to jump-start the development of a group of follicles, although in this case rather than a natural process, the boost is accomplished artificially. After just a few days, the agonist's action will then have the opposite effect, that is, it will suppress both the output of natural FSH and LH. However, if the flare works, the follicles that have begun developing will continue to grow due to the action of the injected FSH. You inject both the agonist and the FSH medication until monitoring shows your follicles are large enough, then you inject hCG and go onto IUI or IVF.

There are many different variations on this theme, however. It turns out that the flare can induce the release of other less beneficial hormones, such as androgen and progesterone, as well as suppress follicle development; these conditions may lead to lower viable pregnancy rates, especially in poor responders. To combat this problem, REs have tried using very low doses of agonists to reduce the detrimental effects and still achieve the flare. Pregnancies have occurred, but rates remain low. Others have tried using a higher dose of the agonist for the first four days, then dropping it to a standard dose, with so-so results. In one study, following 29 cycles using this protocol, the pregnancy rate amounted to 3 percent; one patient took home a baby.

It appears that depending on the clinic and doctor, the agonist flare protocol and the antagonist protocol can achieve similar results, with the antagonist method just slightly better according to recent research. Further testing is underway to determine which will benefit the poor responders of the future.

The Long Protocol

This regimen is used most routinely within the general reproductively challenged population. For the long protocol, agonists are used to quiet or "down-regulate" the ovaries. The GnRH agonist injections begin about a week before your period is expected, and they continue through the stimulation cycle alongside the FSH injections—hence the term *long*. This will essentially turn off your natural secretion of FSH and LH allowing more control of FSH stimulation because natural FSH and LH, are suppressed.

In normal or high responders, too much of a good thing—FSH—can be very bad, and this protocol gives doctors the most control of stimulation. The major concern is *over*-stimulating the ovaries, a condition known as ovarian hyperstimulation syndrome (OHSS). Symptoms can be sudden with too many follicles developing. In rare cases, OHSS can lead to ovarian rupture and stroke. Generally, in older women, poor responders, or those who have had abnormal ovarian reserve test results, OHSS is not a concern.

On the contrary, the long protocol has interfered with the push the ovaries need to wheedle out the most eggs. Using agonists to suppress poor responders may make the ovaries sluggish right when they need some extra punch. Research has consistently shown that rather than the long agonist protocol, either agonist flare protocols or the antagonist protocol is more beneficial for older women and poor responders. A study involving patients who failed the long protocol showed major improvement with the flare protocol—pregnancy rates jumped from 0 to 30 percent in the same patients. Another recent study showed cycle cancellation rates due to poor response dropped substantially using the antagonist protocol, compared to the long protocol. Using the long method, nearly 32 percent of the cycles had to be canceled because of *no response*, whereas when the same patients underwent the antagonist protocol, only 7 percent were canceled. All 63 patients had failed previous long protocols, but with the antagonist method, seven pregnancies resulted, including one set of twins.

Other Variations on These Themes

Some clinicians have enlisted and studied the use of oral contraceptives (OC or OCP in the medical literature, or birth control pill), along with these protocols. Most research has shown that taking OC during the cycle before the stimulation cycle is effective for increasing the numbers of follicles that develop and improving ongoing pregnancy rates. In normal responders, OC have resulted in a pregnancy rate of slightly more than 40 percent. In poor responders the outcomes have also been impressive after pretreatment with OC.

Recent data have shown this is true on either the flare protocol or the antagonist protocol compared to women who did not take OC. In one study using the agonist flare regimen, the pregnancy outcome was 40 percent with OC compared to 33 percent without. In another study, using the antagonist protocol, 1,365 poor responders produced significantly more eggs using OC, putting them in the normal responder range; they also had far fewer cycles canceled. Predicted poor responders using OC showed a high pregnancy rate at 48 percent, whereas without the pretreatment only 37 percent achieved pregnancy.

There are just a couple more variations with which you should at least be familiar. First, some clinicians have used Clomid in combination with FSH drugs. One study showed this mixture increases FSH production, but there was no documented benefit to egg production or fertilization rate. Another earlier study (1995) showed some benefit using Clomid in a select group of patients who had failed previous cycles on other protocols. One of the authors says he still uses this method on occasion, but admits it's a pure guess as to whether it will work.

Another popular approach for potential poor responders is to start treatment on a *good* FSH cycle. The research is mixed on this method, but REs who will go to bat for borderline cases will make the extra effort to test FSH on day two or three on consecutive cycles to find the lowest level and start treatment immediately with the hopes of achieving the best results.

Finally, you might wonder, whether stimulating a cycle longer or adding more FSH can force more eggs into service. Studies have shown that in either case, *more* medication actually decreases success rates. According to recent data, the optimal duration of FSH stimulation is five days; between five and 10 days, there is about a 10-percent drop in pregnancy rate, but further stimulation causes a dramatic drop to essentially zero. As far as upping the dose of FSH beyond 450 IUs, it doesn't seem to work. Think of the FSH injections as stepping on the gas peddle to stimulate your ovaries' engine. If your ovaries are cruising along at 40 mph, and all of a sudden the medications floor it to 90 mph, you should get to your destination in record time, and produce lots of follicles. However, if the engine is ready to fizzle anyway, and your body is already *naturally* producing high levels of FSH—that is, pushing the pedal to the metal—then the extra medication will have little effect.

It's a Jungle out There

Your head may be spinning right about now. But take heart, because most of what is presented you will not find anywhere other than the medical literature. I have tried to provide an overview for women whose decline in fertility will be the most challenging to even the best REs. I hope this information will arm you with the knowledge to advocate for yourself if you either have to, or want to try, ART. It is vitally important that anyone entering treatment understand when it comes to age-compromised fertility, ART is truly more *art* than science. As one top RE once said, "Sometimes I feel like a jungle guide. I can lead patients along what we think might be the best routes, but there are always surprises—some delightful, some traumatic."

Denied Treatment, Failed Treatment, or if You've Had Enough

If you are fortunate to have unlimited resources, or live in a state where fertility treatment is covered, you can likely continue to try repeated stimulated cycles, despite your poor prognosis. However, sometimes after even the first peek at your biological clock via ovarian reserve testing, the prospects are so poor that the clinic may refuse to treat you. Also, if you've tried repeated cycles with varied stimulated protocols for IVF and failed, your RE may strongly discourage further treatment using your own eggs. In addition, after going through the rigors of ART, and experiencing recurring failure and its heart-wrenching disappointment, *you* may decide there must be another way.

The good news is there are other routes to a child, either without the stress of ART, or at least with much better odds of a viable pregnancy. The first step is reaching this crossroads and seriously deciding to look down another path. This can prove easier said than done because it means giving up your genetic heritage. In my case, I had a little help—my insurance company refused to cover IVF with my own eggs. This was devastating to me given I had failed three IUI cycles, endured two difficult miscarriages, and was anticipating IVF would be the magic bullet. We were ready to pay out of pocket for our chance at IVF, but had a change of heart as soon as my doctor said, "Cara, we can do whatever you want, but your odds are 1, maybe 3 percent. You might as well put your $15,000 on a roulette wheel."

As hard as that was to hear, he was right. However, knowing the decision was up to me, and also trusting his expertise, I was able to take the first step down another road toward my second child. Your experience may be entirely different. Most couples live in states where fertility treatment is not covered. If you are faced with next to zero odds, and are ready to take out another mortgage on your house for IVF with your own eggs, it might be a good idea to take a step back and asses your feelings about parenthood, and whether your finances would be better placed toward your eventual child's education or fun vacations, rather than incredibly poor chances of his or her conception. It's critical to assess your financial resources so you can consider other costly options, such as donor eggs, or adoption, in the event that you continue to be unsuccessful with your own eggs.

Typically, if you are faced with incredibly poor chances with IVF using your own eggs, or you can't find a clinic that will treat you with such poor odds, and you decide you still want a child, you are looking at four basic roads you can take: continuing to try on your own *naturally*, using donor eggs from a younger woman, pursuing adoption, or trying on your own while pursuing either of the other two options.

Trying on Your Own With or Without Pursuing Other Options

Isn't it ironic that you start out doing it the "old-fashioned" way, and after you've been hit with the biggest guns medicine has to offer, and failed, your best odds are getting back to nature once again. Remember the gas pedal analogy? If your body already has plenty of

FSH surging, injecting more of it isn't going to do much. As for doing IVF on top of adding what would likely be useless medication to your already revved up system, my doctor says, "You're eggs are not going to feel any better if we take them out and stick them in a dish." The reasoning is that if most of your eggs are like little old ladies, there may be one that can still get the job done, but it probably won't make any difference whether it gets plucked out of your ovary and plopped onto a petri dish. In fact, in it's feeble state, it might be able to perform better in a more natural environment.

Every RE has cases where women have stopped treatment and have become pregnant thanks to candle light rather than surgical light. Many of these cases are in older women. Some are well into their 40s with high FSH.

Andrea is a great example. She began treatment at 31 and succeeded following several miscarriages, and surgery—on her *ninth* IUI. She had her first daughter at 35. Figuring the treatment had solved her problem, she waited 18 months before trying for her second child, and quickly realized she should try IVF. After repeated failures, doctors told her that her age was now playing a role and eventually she turned to donor egg. However, after two attempts with different donors, weeks of acupuncture treatments, and other alternative therapies, nearly eight years later, she still hadn't conceived again. Finally, she called it quits and began exploring adoption. Four months after her last failed donor egg treatment cycle, at age 43, she got pregnant on her own. She still asks herself, "Why did this one stick, why didn't this one miscarry, why did this one happen after treatment, who knows? I don't regret going through all the treatment, because it certainly could have helped. Either way, it is truly a miracle."

Nicki, a casting agent in the Boston area, went through IVF to conceive her first son. She went back to IVF for her second, but failed. Lo and behold, at 42 she got pregnant again—not during, but following treatment. She believes all the ART she went through trying to conceive both times definitely had an impact.

Every RE I interviewed agreed that fertility treatment can have a positive effect on the reproductive system, and may aid in *natural* conception. Dr. Alan DeCherney, noted reproductive endocrinologist, author of several textbooks and textbook chapters, as well as editor in chief of the medical journal *Fertility and Sterility*, confirms,

"You are more fertile in a resting cycle that occurs following a treated cycle. There is some revved up response, some overlap. Many patients get pregnant this way."

One word of warning: if you are not successful, there will come a time when you will run out of steam. Depending on your emotional stamina, failure month after month, or worse, with repeated miscarriages, can completely zap romance. Sex can become drudgery, and mechanical. My husband finally said sarcastically, "I feel like a dancing bear. Just flip the switch, and I'll do my thing." He got tired of the calendar determining when we would have sex. I had more will power to continue, but certainly wasn't enjoying the neverending month to month amusement park ride—it lifted you up only to bring you crashing down, over and over again. Eventually, I decided it would be best for everyone to get off this stomach-churning, emotion-whipping whirlwind. Still, it requires a lot of courage to leave your genetics behind, and take that turn toward a more hopeful, and effective way to bring home a child.

Choosing Donor Egg

Many more couples than you might think are choosing this route. The latest published statistics from the CDC show nearly 11,000 embryos resulting from donor eggs were transferred in 2001. And it's not just older women, according to licensed social worker and infertility expert, Peg Beck, "There are people doing donor egg at 32, 33, 34. It's not just 38 to 45 or 50. There are people who were fertile at 28 to 29, and they just decline more rapidly; many of these younger women opt for donor egg." The advantages are obvious, the CDC data reveals, on average, nearly half of the fresh embryo transfers resulted in live births, and nearly a third of the *frozen* transfers became take-home babies. These rates are better than the national averages for all women attempting IVF with non-donor eggs. That same year, the CDC reported that 89 percent of clinics in the United States offer donor egg services, making the option more accessible than ever before.

For women whose clocks have little or no ticking left, using donor eggs might be compared to cleaning the clock and replacing it with new working parts. In fact, you can take an antique grandmother clock that hasn't worked in years, replace the old gears with newer ones, and she'll crank right up! That's the beauty of donor egg. It doesn't matter if you are menopausal; if you've got most of the essential parts to make a baby, you can—you simply need a single tiny critical piece of machinery to set the process in motion. That part is a younger donor egg.

Aside from the great boost in odds of success, women like the idea that they can maintain their role as caretaker and foreman of the baby-making process. From the beginning, I thought of this in terms of building a beautiful home—you ask someone else to provide the blueprint, but you are in charge of every aspect of the construction, exterior design, landscaping, and every detail of the decorating. With that in mind, you might decide, as I did, that the actual blueprint must have some basic qualities, but what matters most is taking charge, and taking great care of the rest of the process.

Another great feature of this option is that from the moment of fertilization, the baby is *yours*. It will always have a genetic connection to your husband, and everyone in his family, and if you have other genetic children, he or she is genetically related to them. Also, for some women, it is a chance to defy a failed clock. If you are healthy, and want a child, but Mother Nature is preventing you, now you can exercise your ability to create another life, whether Darwin likes it or not.

However, this option has its drawbacks too. Some women find it too strange or high tech. It is also not yet well understood or accepted as a social norm. You may feel uncomfortable explaining your decision to older grandparents, brothers or sisters, extended family, or friends. Those who are uneasy also worry about whether to, or how to, tell the child. Experience from sperm donation and adoption show it is better to explain to children how they came into the world.

In addition, the process of finding a donor can be daunting. Most clinics have their own volunteer program, but the wait can often be years rather than months, and generally, the clinic usually decides whose eggs you will use. Most REs will encourage couples to find a relative or a friend to donate. However, this is not always possible or desirable. Some women search for their own non-relative donor by advertising on the Web, in local papers, or college papers. This is time intensive and can be difficult, because you must interview potential donors, and ask many personal questions. The newest option is hiring an agency to find your donor. Several privately owned donor egg-matching services have flourished in the past few years. These agencies charge from $3,500 to $10,000, not including the donor fee. Many search nationwide, and can usually help anyone, anywhere. There may be additional travel expenses, but it's often possible to locate a donor in your area, making logistics easier and lightening the financial load.

As you can imagine, the fees involved in finding and using an egg donor can climb rather quickly. The main costs are the donor; the agency fee; legal fees; travel expenses; her lost wages; her medical expenses, including screening tests not covered by her insurance; all of her and your medications; and the treatment. Just to give you a ballpark figure, donors' fees start at about $4,000, but climb to the stratosphere. Donors have become savvy in recent years, and have begun charging upwards of $15 to $20 thousand or more, depending on their education and appearance.

This is the ugly side of egg donation, and it poses a major ethical dilemma for some couples. They feel that donors should offer this gift free of charge. Others, including experts such as Ellen Glazer, a licensed social worker specializing in third-party reproduction and adoption, also author of several books on various related topics, says she has clients who refuse to pay a cent to an egg donor. Glazer understands these concerns, but also appreciates the commitment the donor makes. "I am troubled by anything more than a minimal payment for egg donation, though I think a donor should be compensated."

If women want to donate to help a couple, they should ask for reasonable compensation for their time and discomfort, not for their genes. Couples who are willing, and in some cases advertising to pay exorbitant fees to donors are fueling this practice, ultimately undermining the altruistic idea of *donating* eggs to a those in need. In addition, it is illegal to sell any kind of body tissue or organs, but by charging outrageous fees based on genetics, or Ivy League status, that is exactly what these young women are doing. The fee should be relatively standard based on cost of living, and it should represent compensation for making and keeping appointments; learning how to prepare and inject the medications; following the doctor's instructions; and for the discomfort of the egg retrieval. All donors go through the same process, and should be paid appropriately and consistently for their services only—legally and morally, it should have nothing to do with their eggs or the genes they carry.

The most important drawback to using a donor is that there are no guarantees. Remember, about 50 of every 100 women who undergo the procedure fail on the fresh cycle. Generally, a young donor will produce many eggs, so you will likely have extra embryos to freeze for more tries. Still, while many women have success with a frozen cycle (approximately 30 percent), most will not. Failure after coming this far can prove an emotional crisis. For this reason, many who choose this option will approach it with plan "B" already in place. That way, couples can move on, without too much trauma if this final ART attempt fails.

Choosing Adoption

Couples who fail donor egg will often opt for adoption; in fact, some begin their adoption research in conjunction with their donor search. Plenty of others, however, choose adoption over egg donation to realize their dream of parenthood. These couples either shy away from the high-tech nature of donor egg, or simply prefer the comfort of a more traditional route to family building. Glazer says, "With adoption there are no ethical questions, there are no moral issues at all."

Adoption is socially well accepted; there is no dilemma around who to tell or what to tell. Couples often feel it's incredibly rewarding to give an unwanted child a home, and a chance. This is especially true with international adoptions where countless children grow up in orphanages if they are not adopted. Domestically, there are more families wanting to adopt than there are babies.

Many adoptive parents report their experience is wonderful, full of joy and fulfillment. Mary and Mike failed with donor egg and wasted no time turning to adoption. The happy couple received their baby in less than a year, and said they wished they had considered adoption sooner.

However, adoptive parents also say that the process, like donor egg, often has its obstacles. Kate, a highly respected Ivy League university professor who gave up on fertility treatment is still trying to adopt a son after several years of effort and *four* failed international adoptions. You would think that she and her husband, also a university professor and author, might have a little leverage—not so. Their first attempt ended in disappointment when a birth parent changed

138

her mind, then months later decided to put the child up for adoption again. Kate had begun pursuing another child, but because she was so bonded with the first, decided to try for him instead. Ultimately, the judge overseeing the case in Chile denied their request. Then two more South American adoptions fell through due to severe medical issues with the children.

Other potential roadblocks to keep in mind include the high cost and travel expenses. Today, it's not unusual to spend $30 to $40 thousand per child for a domestic or international adoption, depending on the agency, the country, and the complications that may arise. However, unlike donor egg, a portion of the cost is tax-deductible, and many large companies offer adoption benefits. Experts in adoption also counsel couples on the possible health issues they may encounter with infants and children from the adoptive population. Though this is a difficult topic, it is imperative that families are aware so they can be prepared to deal with the potential needs of their children. The most common problems are attention deficit hyperactivity disorder (ADHD), developmental delays, and learning disabilities. Many families are more than willing to adopt a child with special needs or disabilities, others have trouble coming to terms with such difficulties.

Child-Free, or Stopping at One or Two

Some couples who come to the end of the ART road focus their energies elsewhere. Psychologists say this can be a very difficult decision, especially following the disappointments of fertility treatment, or failed adoptions. Peg Beck counsels clients who are struggling with the issue. "The right decision is not always without pain, and so it can be very sad. It can require a period of grief, but if couples get through it, many of them find something new and wonderful in their lives instead. Some people find a new career, some retire early and buy a yacht, some discover other children that are very special in their lives." The advantage of this choice is you have almost limitless options to pour your time, energy, and financial resources. While the joy of parenthood is a special gift, living child-free and devoting time and attention to other children or a special cause can also bring much happiness.

Couples who already have one or two children are more apt to forego donor egg or adoption, and focus on the child or children they already have. Given the costs involved, it is sometimes difficult to justify spending tens of thousands of dollars, and weeks and months of effort on trying to have another, rather than on the needs and desires of the family that already exists. However, often women in particular, are caught off guard by how traumatic it is to be unable to have a *second* child. Even a woman who never wanted children may find the pleasures and joy of bringing another life into the world can be so intense that she feels even more strongly about having a second child than she did about having the first.

The trouble is, with age-related fertility problems, women are stunned when they discover they have run out of time. If, for some reason, they are unable to pursue donor egg or adoption, the lack of control or choice may bring on regret and heartache that can last a lifetime. With some effort and counseling, it is possible to work through this loss. Hopefully the information you have gathered will allow *you* to make decisions that will help prevent such an emotionally and financially draining experience.

ADJUST YOUR THINKING

6.

I'd really like to have another child, but figure I'll wait a couple of years. I have time—hey, Joan Lunden had twins at 52!

—Diedre, age 37, mother of IVF baby Peter, age 1

I had a woman bring me in an article from Glamour, and say, "But if so and so can do it, I can do it, she's older than I am. Why are you telling me at 48 that I can't have a baby when this person did it?"

—Dr. Marcelle Cedars, reproductive endocrinologist

They seek the publicity and yet they tell half a story, and the half they are telling is destructive to other people. I think they should just shut up. If you want privacy, then shut up!

—Peg Beck, infertility counselor

Hear This...

Is the message clear? This chapter is right out of your high school critical thinking lesson: don't believe everything you hear or read. In this case it could overly promote the sense of security you may have with your fertility, or at least unrealistically boost your confidence in the current capabilities of reproductive medicine.

Sometimes one of the greatest obstacles to having your own genetic child is the general comfort you may have with your fertility. Like you, I became an adult during a time when birth control was a nonissue. Today we continue to embrace the option, and month after month, we go on with our lives, pursuing our careers, never really thinking about whether we can, in fact, get pregnant. I'd bet you are pretty sure you would become pregnant immediately if you're not extremely careful with your birth control method. At some point, however, this becomes a dangerous assumption.

After age 35, many women finally get a peek at their aging biological clocks when they walk into a reproductive medicine clinic for the first time and get the results of their first FSH test. They are shocked and saddened to learn their once vibrant, efficient clock is now a slow, ineffective timepiece. Women can feel cheated, angry, and in some cases very guilty over a previous abortion, because for more than a decade now, they've received so many positive messages in the media regarding older mothers and the miracles accomplished with reproductive medicine. While in my 30s and very single, every time I saw an interview with an older celebrity mom holding her baby, I thought, "Gee, that's great, if I run out of time, I'll just go to a fertility clinic." It was nearly 10 years ago, but I remember one magazine cover in particular—a smiling celebrity mom alongside the headline "Twins at 45!" I never bought the magazine, never even opened it. But that positive message imprinted in my mind. It was all I needed to know. It gave me hope, it helped mask the ticking sound, and it blinded me to reality.

Miracle Babies?

We hear about them sometimes weekly or at least monthly. Celebrities having babies later in life—in their late 30s, mid-40s, even in their 50s. Sometimes they hire a gestational carrier, also known as a surrogate carrier, which essentially means a woman who gestates a child for a couple, but has no genetic connection to it. Often, if a surrogate is used, it is mentioned in the story, but so far I have not seen any celebrity reveal in a major publication or talk show that she also used *donor eggs*. However, according to several reproductive endocrinologists who have either treated celebrities, or know the doctors that did: they do.

Just to set the record straight here. Celebrities are not the only ones. Thousands of women opt to use donor eggs every year. In 2001 the CDC reported 11 percent of all ART cycles used embryos created from donor eggs and a husband's sperm. That's a total of 10,750 transfers using donor eggs rather than the mother's eggs. That year, on average, half of the transfers using fresh embryos rather than frozen, resulted in babies. Also it's important to realize that this number rises substantially every year.

The difference is, the other 99.99 percent of these women do not don magazine covers, chat with Larry King on primetime cable TV, or drop by network morning shows to chat about mid-life motherhood. Don't get me wrong, I think it's wonderful for famous women to use the media to promote motherhood, and share their stories about their struggles with infertility. What is unfair and misleading is not sharing the *whole* story, if indeed they did use donor eggs. What is even worse is to outright deny the fact, if asked.

It is not impossible to have a child later in life, but it is safe to say, it is *next to* impossible—especially with treatment—for any particular woman over 43. That's right, 43! A recent study published in the medical journal *Fertility and Sterility* underscores just how rare *natural* births are during mid-40s or later. Results show that in a population of women over 45 that does not use contraception, natural pregnancies and deliveries amount to a mere 0.2 percent! The study also reveals that the women who were most likely to have children after 45 had *six* or more previous pregnancies! Researchers say they are not sure whether having so many pregnancies delays the natural decline in fertility, or whether these women simply possess a genetic trait that allows their ovaries to age more slowly than the rest of ours. Either way, the bottom line is that natural pregnancies are extremely uncommon after the mid-40s, so those in the media spotlight in this age category who deny they used donor eggs when they did, or share their stories but leave out this part of it, give false hope to millions of women.

Parade of Celebrity Midlife Babies

Of course, regardless of how the baby was initially created, it is wonderful news for any couple to become parents, and it's especially happy when one of our favorite celebrities is successful in this life-affirming endeavor. For some reason, we are even more joyous when we hear that an older celebrity mom or couple has given birth. Perhaps it is because we have come to know them over a longer period of time, or we innately know that it wasn't easy at their age, or perhaps we feel they must have wanted this child intensely because they waited so long, and in many cases needed treatment of one kind or another to have the child. Whatever the reason, we truly revel in their happiness.

Besides, it's good news, and we feel good when we hear Geena Davis is 48 and having twins; Peri Gilpin (Roz on *Frasier*) became a mom at 42 thanks to a gestational surrogate; at 52, after fertility treatments, and finally with help from a gestational surrogate, Joan Lunden became the proud mother of twins and her three previous daughters now in their teens and 20s are thrilled; Susan Sarandon had her third child at 45; Jane Seymour, also at 45, had twins after struggling with infertility; and Cheryl Tiegs became a mother for the second time at 52 with the help of a gestational surrogate. The list goes on.... Mimi Rogers, Madonna, Beverly D'Angelo, Caroline Taylor (James's wife), and Deidre Hall, all had babies in their 40s.

But given the ever-expanding list, you have to wonder whether there is something in their genes that not only provided them with talent, but a biological clock to-die-for as well. Are they truly super-women? Do their eggs have a longer shelf life or do they start off with more to begin with? According to Michael Soules, M.D., former president of ASRM and director of the department of Obstetrics and Gynecology, Reproductive Medicine/Infertility at the University of Washington School of Medicine, the answer is none of the above. "Celebrity status does not give somebody a better biological clock. It doesn't make sense that they're defying biology. Some have to be using donor eggs. That's fine, that's an option." Soules says to just do the menopause versus infertility math. If the extreme upper limit for normal menopause is age 58, and you backtrack 10 years to the predictable sudden fertility decline, then there will be a few women who will have reasonable fertility at 48. "But you're talking less than 5 percent of the population. Could it happen? Yes. Is it likely? No," says Soules.

144

Alan DeCherney, M.D., reproductive endocrinologist, Editor-in-Chief of the medical journal Fertility and Sterility, professor at the UCLA School of Medicine, and author of several medical textbooks, is even more blunt by saying, "Donor eggs. They're donor eggs without a doubt. I know that for certain." DeCherney says the use of donor eggs is understood in reproductive medicine circles, and thinks celebrity moms who use donor eggs should get over their reluctance about the issue—if they want to go public with their baby news. "It's silly. People know," he says.

Twin Stories, Two Approaches

On the evening of July 14, 2000, Cheryl Tiegs and her former husband Rod Stryker appeared on CNN's *Larry King Live* to talk about the new additions to their family: twin boys. They discussed parenthood, the struggles they had trying to get pregnant with treatment, and the surrogate that they ultimately used that made the difference. But when King asked Tiegs directly if she used donor eggs, she denied it, and essentially said that because she took such good care of herself for so long, that at 52, it is possible to produce a baby with your own eggs. Tiegs went on to say that she wouldn't recommend waiting, because, "it was not an easy process, but it certainly was possible." As proof, she mentioned the California woman who at the time became the oldest to have a baby at nearly 64, but failed to point out that this woman used donor eggs. In fact, that truth became part of the highly publicized national story, because she was the first to succeed *with* donor eggs at such an advanced age.

A little later in the broadcast, Stryker alluded to their problem as an age-related issue. He talked about even healthy women running out of time, and finding out they can't get pregnant "with the normal means." Just for the record, when advanced age is an issue, even in menopausal women, peer-reviewed scientific data has shown time and again, it is an egg problem rather than a uterus problem.

Finally, a caller who went through many IVF cycles then turned to donor egg to have her child, tried to pin Tiegs down just one more time. "There's no documented [IVF] cases of any woman getting pregnant with her own eggs past 46...." Tiegs replied, "Well, then I'm on the record." In every media account of this story, Tiegs has said they were *her* eggs. Most recently, media accounts have centered on the couple's divorce. Stryker was awarded full custody of the twin boys.

145

Two years later, Larry King sat across from another celebrity mom, who was also having twins at age 52 through a gestational surrogate. This time it was Joan Lunden, former cohost of *Good Morning America*, and producer/host on A&E. Lunden immediately revealed that they had tried IVF for several years before turning to a surrogate. She provided no further details. However, she did explain that they used a *gestational* surrogate rather than a traditional surrogate, making clear that their surrogate had no genetic connection to the implanted embryos/fetuses. Here's a bit of the exchange:

> King: "And the embryo comes from?"
> Lunden: "It can be your egg and sperm, it can be a donor. And I think that's something that's personal between each couple and it's your private business.
> King: "But that's your business whether it's Jeff's sperm and your egg. That's personal."
> Lunden: "That's our business."

In another more recent interview with Deborah Norville on MSNBC, Lunden's reaction was even more pointed:

> Norville: "So let me get this straight, so it was Jeff's sperm...."
> Lunden: "No, you know something, I never, even if I thought that was an appropriate question to answer, which I don't, I think that is a very personal question for each couple, I don't answer it because I don't ever want anyone out there to think, 'Gee, I didn't live up to this,' I couldn't do that, knowing that you don't want to set standards for others."

Here, it sounds as if your *uterus* is the major fertility problem as you age. The medical fact is that in the vast majority of cases, and, in virtually all cases of women nearing or over 50, it is the *eggs*. In fact, medicine has proven that uteruses over 60 years old are capable of carrying a child. The upper age limit for a functioning uterus isn't even known, because ethically, no doctors have dared try to reach it. The fact is plenty of 50-plus women have been able to bear children with their own bodies and younger donor eggs. By talking about the gestational surrogate only, Lunden suggests that in her case, it was the other way around, that her eggs were fine, but her uterus wasn't. At the very least this is confusing from a medical standpoint.

One highly respected reproductive endocrinologist insists women who are in the media spotlight and have used donor eggs, have an obligation to say so. "At that age it's normal. Any woman would be a freak if it were her own eggs. It's that rare."

When Publicity and Personal Lives Clash

Media outlets, which look to celebrities for stories about their personal lives, and the personalities who oblige, have always had a mutually beneficial relationship. The reporters and producers get their stories, and the actors and TV anchors have their names and faces peppered around the nation in all forms of media. In fact, according to TV news talent agent David Ahrendts of the Napoli Management Group, positive publicity about any facet of a public person's life can be critical to continued career success. "If you're talking about a public presenter, if you're talking about a celebrity, if you are talking about a television news anchor, to constantly have that kind of attention can be simply vital."

Given my experience as a TV reporter, I would say it is even more critical for middle-aged women to remain in the public eye as much as possible. Also, let's not forget that in our youth-oriented society, older celebrities (unless you are Barbara Walters!) must strive to remain youthful, on top of their game, and yes, to some extent, sexy! What better way to prove to the public, and those who would hire you, that you are all of these things, than to have a baby! Fertility = youth— does it not?

It is a catch-22 for these women. Their careers dictate the need for media attention, but they also understandably desire to omit some details from their personal stories. However, in this case, the omission can do irreparable harm to other women who believe they can do the same. Leading women to believe they used their own eggs, when in fact they haven't, is destructive—even if it is not the celebrity's intention. Women postpone having children, believing if a role model can have babies at 45 or 52, then they can surely have them at 39 or even 48. Unfortunately, in the majority of cases (and I know from experience), this is not necessarily true.

Unveiling a natural age-related loss of fertility and suffering the perceived negative implications may be a strong motive to remain so reluctant to come out with this choice, but other reasons include the same worries all people have: real privacy issues, and social acceptance. Many couples feel strongly about protecting their children's private lives; many opt to keep this information even from close family and friends. Revealing such details, they fear, could come back to haunt them or their children. For celebrities, these feelings are likely exaggerated exponentially. Add to that the fact that donor egg is yet to become a social norm, and it's hardly a stretch to realize a celebrity believes she could risk a positive story turning negative—instantly.

It is also curious that so many high-profile moms feel it's fine to reveal they used a gestational surrogate. Many promote and celebrate their surrogate carriers, even appearing on magazine covers with them. This kind of enthusiasm no doubt helps the general public feel more comfortable with this reproductive choice. Still, wouldn't people be just as apt to share the joy of giving through egg donation if it is presented just as passionately? Perhaps this is the catch: everyone can relate to carrying and giving birth to a baby, but how many can truly appreciate the egg-donation process? The procedure is very high tech; it involves a younger woman, and it is generally portrayed in the media as a sticky social problem. Again, it makes sense that celebrities would shy away from discussing it, though that doesn't make it right. On the contrary, if it were presented as one of the most profound things a woman can do for another woman and her family, perhaps this image would change.

Medical Truths and Media

Whether it's cancer therapy, diet fads, or reproductive medicine, the stakes are high when passing on any degree of medical information to the public. Though many of these midlife baby stories usually fall under entertainment news rather than medical news, as soon as there is any hint of treatment, the take-home message changes. Ethicists agree that when fertility treatment is involved, and a celebrity wants to go public with her success story, she must be responsible enough to provide the full picture. Paul Wolpe, Ph.D., bioethicist at the University of Pennsylvania School of Medicine contends, "If you are going to get on television and talk about those kinds of things, then you have to be rigorous about what kinds of information you give clearly." But according to Wolpe, only part of the burden for full disclosure rests with the celebrity. He says that print and TV journalists must be vigilant as well. "Absolutely, they should be asking those questions. It's the responsibility of people in the media—who know that the public sees these reports and uses them as information, not just as entertainment—to make sure the public has the correct information."

Some ethicists say, even if the subject of the story shies away from certain details, the reporter should at least provide statistics on donor eggs or other information that will give the public a more accurate perspective on the medical side of the story. Unfortunately, few entertainment reporters are encouraged, or trained, to do this. In the grand scheme of entertainment news, spending time digging up medical details is hardly necessary; simply getting a personality to talk with you is often all that matters.

There are signs, however, that some journalists are doing their homework. *Good Housekeeping*'s cover story following the birth of Lunden's twins reported the story comprehensively, also running a side-bar plainly stating known data:

> ...after age 45, a vast 95 percent of women are unable to conceive on their own. And after 50, virtually all women who give birth, do so with eggs from donors in their 20s or early 30s.

These two medically accurate facts in any story about a midlife baby give a reader or viewer enough information to decide what the take-home message is, regardless of what the celebrity says or doesn't say.

Cracking the Donor Egg Code

Those in reproductive medicine circles, be they REs, patients, or patient advocates, know how to spot a possible donor egg recipient a mile away. The following list of donor egg clues was compiled through dozens of interviews with experts in the field of reproductive endocrinology. Here's what to look for:

- ☺ Age. The older a woman is, the greater the chances that she used donor eggs.
- ☺ Previous ART treatment, especially IVF.
- ☺ Reported miscarriages. They are very common with age-related infertility.

- ☉ Had children previously when younger without any problem.
- ☉ It is a first pregnancy in mid-40s or older.
- ☉ Twins, very common with young viable donated eggs.
- ☉ Gestational surrogate, you know the eggs didn't come from her.

Of course, each of these clues, and even a few combinations, do not necessarily mean a donor was used, but certainly, the more signs, the more you should probably lean toward thinking *donor eggs*. Again, this is protection for you. Don't be mislead, enjoy the news these celebrity older moms impart, be happy for them, and at the same time, be mindful of separating their reported miracle or good fortune from *your* biological clock.

Nevermind Celebrities, What About Your Next-Door Neighbor?

When I was struggling to have another baby, and considering trying to find an egg donor, my home daycare mom said to me as I was dropping off my son, "You should talk to Linda, she's pregnant with twins through a donor." As my son ran off to play with Linda's son Jack (an IVF baby), I thought to myself, *Wow, who would have thought in this little town, at this neighborhood home daycare, I'd find another woman not only thinking about, but actually pregnant after using donor eggs!* I had heard about all the celebrities, and wondered about their use of donor eggs, but after this brief conversation, I was convinced that there are many more people choosing this family-building option than most people realize.

When I finally took the plunge and realistically considered this option, I joined a donor egg support group through Resolve of the Baystate, my local chapter. Upwards of 40 people attended some of these meetings, and many more had already revolved through the group, and had babies. The fact is, this is now a real option for women, and not just much older women. There are plenty of women like me who had a baby near 40, and within a year or two couldn't have another; there are women like Anne who just got married at 39, and has failed several IUI and IVF attempts and may eventually turn to this option; and there are women such as Linda who went through IVF at 35 to have her first, and at 37 with poor egg quality, successfully chose a donor to help her complete her family.

Given that there are really no other options to bear a child once IVF has failed, or indications are so dismal that IVF is no longer a consideration, and the majority of couples *can* have children this way, wouldn't it be best for all of us if we start talking about it? I mentioned earlier that celebrities might be reluctant to reveal this choice because it implies they are "old." On the contrary, doesn't it really only suggest that biology is backward? Any woman who wants to have a child at 40 or 50, is anything but old! Who cares if her ovaries are not with the program!

The fact is, if we were to adopt, nobody would even question our age. For many of us, though, carrying a child, having some kind of genetic and biologic connection to him or her, as we have always planned, is our choice, especially given it is now a real possibility. There are times when I take a moment and think about my donor, and it always brings tears to my eyes. As I sit here trying to finish these last couple of chapters while my daughter wiggles in my belly, I think to myself, *Thank you! Thank you for being an angel who came to my rescue, who has given me the chance to be a mother again, my husband to be a father again, my son the opportunity to be a big brother, by providing us with the tiny single-cell egg that is going to make a new, incredibly loved child possible.* What a gift!

This is what we need to hear from celebrities who can make the cover of magazines, or sit down with Larry King or Deborah Norville for an hour. How about it? If you are the next high-profile older mom who used a donor, would you do us all a favor, and talk about it? Let the world know it's okay, it's a fantastic option, and donors are just as important as surrogates. If setting the record straight for younger women isn't enough motivation, how about doing it for all the donor-created children that are coming into this world? Our children need to know how special they are, how wanted they were, and that there are many others who came into the world in exactly the same way. For the sake of our kids, we need positive donor egg stories, and a celebrity spokeswoman is in a perfect position to do so. Don't think about it, just do it! Please, it is time....

While we wait to see if someone has the courage to be the first, *you* at least now know donor-egg babies are becoming more common, so the next time you hear about a miracle midlife baby, try thinking, *donor egg*, until proven otherwise. That way, you'll most likely be right, and at the very least, you'll remain realistic about your own fertility.

Voices From the Field

Every time a 40- or 50-something high-profile personality announces a pregnancy or birth in the mass media, the first people to feel the effects are reproductive endocrinologists. Their phones start ringing off their hooks. Irate patients call and demand similar treatment, some even accuse their doctors of holding back treatments for their most famous, sophisticated, or rich patients. Clinic directors even report dispatching their staff members to damage-control status. That means answering a flurry of calls from angry patients and reassuring those in for office visits that they are receiving the best care medicine can offer at the moment, regardless of what they hear on the morning news or see on magazine covers.

Misinformation or lack of information in the media has thrown the field of reproductive endocrinology into a tailspin on more than one occasion. A few years back, the then president of the ASRM decided to do something about it. Michael Soules, M.D., initiated the Protect Your Fertility campaign to focus attention on the four best ways to better your chances of having children, if you want them. The campaign raised eyebrows, and became controversial enough that it garnered a tremendous amount of media attention. In fact, the ads themselves, depicting baby bottles and sending the message that unprotected sex, cigarette smoking, being overweight, and getting older can undermine the biological clock, got very little play due to budget constraints, and rejection at venues such as malls and movie theaters.

But the media latched onto the hottest of the four issues: age. Once in the spotlight, the National Organization for Women opposed the campaign and accused the ASRM of using scare tactics to force young women to have babies before they are ready. This just attracted even more media attention. Soules says the media was crucial to getting the message out, especially for such a low budget campaign. "It would have cost us many millions to get that level of exposure if we were buying it."

Others have also added their voices to the chorus of fertility gurus echoing the same message. Zev Rosenwaks, M.D., director at the Center for Reproductive Medicine and Infertility at Weill Medical College at Cornell, wrote an op-ed piece for the *New York Times* that took aim directly at dispelling beliefs that medicine can help women have "genetic children" whenever they like. He writes, "…The media have made a best seller out of the freshly minted fiction of 'rewinding the biological clock.' We can't and we haven't." He goes on to state in no uncertain terms, "Women who contemplate postponing childbearing should know that they may not be able to conceive with their own eggs."

The American Infertility Association has tried to push the issue into the spotlight as often as possible. This organization has put out brochures, written articles, and even conducted a survey to prove how misinformed the public is regarding fertility. The results showed only one person in more than 12,000 answered the questions correctly.

Still, with all the information that pops up from time to time, many women remain either in the dark about their fertility, they buy into the celebrity announcements, or convince themselves, "I'm in great shape, never smoked, and have regular periods—it won't happen to me." Robert Stillman, M.D., clinic director and member of the ASRM Protect Your Fertility committee, believes women can be resistant to receiving this information. "If you hear a message that fits with the message you want to hear, it resonates a lot more than it would if you were hearing a message that's against it. You would reject that. We're giving the counterstream message and people don't necessarily want to hear it." However, he says as long as the information gets out, women will assimilate it whether they want to or not. "You may fight initially, but you've integrated it. I think that's what we are trying to do—get the message out and let people do with it what they will." This was Soules's intention in the first place. "If you are informed, you shouldn't ignore it; you may decide to act on it, or be able to act on it, but make a conscious decision, and don't let life make it for you." Ditto.

NOT NECESSARILY SCIENCE FICTION

7.

Within decades we are going to be able to use any cell in the body and create a sperm or egg cell from it. We will be able to do incredible things with manipulating germ tissue, and it will become so routine that the question of who should be able do it won't even be relevant.

—Paul Wolpe, Ph.D., bioethicist,
University of Pennsylvania School of Medicine

Science in the Spotlight

Science has the ability to both amaze and horrify. Unlike most human endeavors, once scientific research has produced results, there is no turning back. You can destroy a painted canvas, and you can discard the notes to a symphony, but you cannot put knowledge back in the beaker, or pitch it out with used pipettes. All you can do is put it to use either by applying it, or exploiting it to gain further understanding. This truth has produced some of the most astounding breakthroughs in the field of human reproduction, as well some of the most feared.

A little more than 25 years ago, the first successful in vitro fertilization was performed in the United Kingdom, three years later the United States had its first test-tube baby. Since then a host of technologies have given rise to more reproductive options: embryo freezing provides additional opportunities to become parents; intracytoplasmic sperm injection (ICSI) can now make a man a dad even if he has barely any sperm; preimplantation genetic diagnosis (PGD) allows doctors to screen for genetic defects in embryos using a single embryonic cell, preventing devastating chromosomal and genetic diseases; and using donor eggs plus synchronized drug protocols, have essentially turned back the biological clock to help older, even postmenopausal women become mothers.

It wasn't that long ago when visionaries could only speculate on these possibilities. Now they are daily realities inside reproductive medicine clinics across much of the world. Given the strides in such a relatively short period of time, it is reasonable and tempting to ask, what's next?

The Final Frontier

Though ART has advanced tremendously in the last quarter century, there remain several fundamental questions yet to be answered. None seem as pressing as those focusing on the basic mechanisms of the biological clock. Even some of the most elementary truisms in this arena are now under scrutiny, being questioned to the point where basic biology textbooks may have to be rewritten. Make no mistake, when it comes to the state of knowledge about the reproductive life cycle, there remain many more questions than answers. Science, it appears, has yet to crack the code of the biological clock—what triggers it to begin ticking in fetal life; what causes massive amounts of cell death after birth; whether human ovaries contain stem cells that produce new eggs after birth, and, if so, why eggs die throughout the ensuing five decades; exactly what happens to eggs after age 35 to render them incapable of creating a child; and what can be done to halt the relentless process *before* the ticking stops?

Some researchers are working to answer these essential questions—questions that could provide treatment options in the future. Others are in the process of developing medical technologies for women

156

currently suffering with premature ovarian/clock failure or facing a rusting clock precisely when they have decided to start or complete their families. Though the federal government has stepped in and halted certain techniques, research is marching onward, albeit slowly, and eventually experts believe there will be many new options for women who want to preserve their fertility, energize their withering eggs, or stave off menopause.

Why Tinker With Mother Nature?

The Numbers and the Need

Surely the vast majority of women who attempt to start their families at a young age will have little trouble doing so. But it is clear that more women than ever before are waiting to start their families, encountering problems, and then flocking to reproductive medicine clinics in unprecedented numbers. At the same time, the majority of these women are facing a life crisis they never anticipated. The CDC statistics on ART have consistently shown that more often than not, women of all ages are unsuccessful at achieving pregnancy even with technology. Success rates plummet to less than 20 percent and sometimes even less than 10 percent for women in their late 30s, falling to near zero beginning in the early 40s.

The CDC has been publicly reporting records of all ART procedures in the United States since 1995. Indeed, 2001 (the latest year with published statistics) produced the greatest number of babies ever born through assisted reproductive technology—and most of the technology was administered to women 35 and over. Since the mid-90s, the number of ART cycles performed in women over age 35 using fresh non-donor embryos has jumped dramatically from 26,773 to 41,118. Also, during the same time frame, the numbers of women opting to use donor eggs more than doubled. In 1995 the CDC reported just 4,783 cycles using fresh embryos from donor eggs, but in 2001 the number jumped to more than 12,000 cycles. Most of the women who used their own eggs (70 to 80 percent) were between 34 and 39 years old, and the vast majority of women over 39 used donor eggs to create their embryos. These women generally chose donor eggs not first, but as a last resort.

These statistics, however, represent the tip of the iceberg—that is, only the most motivated of hopeful mothers. A recent study published in the journal *Fertility and Sterility* showed that even when the top-level procedure (IVF) is covered by insurance, many women drop out of treatment. Researchers in Sweden followed 450 couples, and found that more than half discontinued treatment before they had exhausted their *covered* IVF cycles. Most stated their reason as psychological burden, or poor prognosis. Essentially, even though they could have continued trying, they gave up. In a related article in the same publication, Alice Domar, Ph.D., founder of the Mind/Body Center at Boston IVF, and an expert on infertility's psychological factors, isn't surprised by these results, she proposes that "the patient's mental health be considered an integral component of her infertility care... her level of anxiety and depression and her ability to cope during crises should be assessed." Domar's earlier research revealed that psychologically, women experience infertility much the same way cancer, cardiac, and hypertension patients suffer with their diseases. In fact, their anxiety and depression scores were strikingly similar.

Domar's investigations also show that psychological intervention, in the form of counseling or support groups, not only helped patients cope, it helped them become pregnant! If infertility is as devastating as other conditions where medical as well as psychological treatments are encouraged, and are effective, shouldn't those experiencing infertility have the same access to such care? New technologies, medications, or other methods that can postpone infertility courtesy of the biological clock, would provide more control over personal lives and health for younger women anticipating a delay in motherhood.

The Career Conundrum

In today's society, many women, especially college educated, career inspired women wait until their early to mid-30s to begin thinking about having children. It would be trite to say, "Don't wait," because today that kind of simplistic solution is pointless. Many professional fields are less than sympathetic to women who want families, especially while they are still climbing the corporate ladder, working toward tenure, or striving for partnership in a law practice. In most cases, fertility has already begun to wane during these most critical years in a hard fought, educationally demanding, competitive career. Even when policies are in place to help women who have children, many report taking advantage of such programs amounts to professional suicide.

A tenured professor at a prestigious university, Paula, can relate. She could have delayed applying for tenure after her son was born, but she reasoned there would be less competition earlier, so she jumped on the fast track, and succeeded. In the highly competitive field of academics, it's no secret that women are wary of such programs, she says, "Universities are accommodating in that they typically allow one extra year per child for tenure, but at some institutions, the word of mouth is, if you take that year, it's the kiss of death."

After struggling with secondary infertility for several years, she now counsels her aspiring students on the biological clock, family planning, as well as career planning. "I lecture them, often during meetings. I ask them, 'What age do think is the latest you can have children?' And it's always 40. Then I tell them, 'You cannot be thinking 40, you have to be thinking 30.'" She also provides even more sobering anecdotes, "Women who have children before they're postdocs or before they get their first job, drop out of science. If you have a child after you're an assistant professor, you've already landed that first position, you stay in it. But it is brutal to women because the time that you need to be starting up a lab, writing your proposals, working literally 12 to 14 hour days, is your child-bearing years, so many never make it."

Reproductive medicine clinics see a steady flow of women who have either decided on their own, or with their husbands or partners, that they have achieved enough financial stability to start a family, and/or finally met Mr. Right—only to find they've run out of time. "It's a huge problem. It's a large portion of my practice," says Bradford Kolb, M.D., a reproductive endocrinologist at the Huntington Reproductive Center in Pasadena, California. "The number of people having infertility problems in their 20s and 30s is the same as it was probably 50 years ago, but what's changed is *when* people are having kids. Well over half my patients are there because of age-related factors."

Unfortunately, only a few in this group are lucky enough, have the financial resources, or can maintain the stamina, to be successful with IVF; the rest must opt to use donor eggs, pursue adoption, or reconcile their yearning for a child. Further advances might surely provide additional, more desirable options.

Cancer Treatments and the Clock

There is no question that there is one group that desperately needs more options to preserve fertility. They are among the 120,000 men and women under the age of 45 diagnosed with cancer each year. Twelve thousand of these patients are children under the age of 19. If they require chemotherapy, radiation, or any combination of treatments, the vast majority can expect to become infertile within months or a few years following these life-saving protocols. What's worse, most of them are never informed of this unfortunate consequence of treatment, and are devastated once they realize that there were options available to them for having children after the treatment left them infertile. For example, men have been able to freeze their sperm with tremendous success for decades.

Today, there are options for women, but all are still considered investigational. Lindsay Nohr, founder of Fertile Hope, a fertility advocacy and resource organization for cancer patients, says more needs to be done. "I think research in this area is tremendously important, and it benefits cancer patients, but it also benefits society at large. Whether you're back is against the wall and you can't have children because you are about to undergo cancer treatment, or because you are turning 40, either way you are in a predicament. If there were a way to preserve your fertility, you should be able to take advantage of it."

Science of the Deep Freeze

It's been more than 200 years since Italian researchers first decided to freeze animal sperm; and more than 60 years since scientists froze then thawed human sperm, and peered into their microscopes with amazement when they saw wiggling, forward-swimming, reincarnated gametes. Today, freezing sperm is easy, efficient, effective, and inexpensive. With the advent of IVF, it wasn't long before embryologists decided to test the deep freeze on extra embryos. The first birth from a frozen embryo took place in 1984, and since, tens of thousands of children have been born. For many undergoing intensive ART, having embryos on ice means a second or third chance for a child, just

160

in case the fresh cycle fails. All these frozen embryos, however, also pose an ethical, moral, and sometimes legal dilemma for couples once they have a child, and no longer need them. Many can't bring themselves to destroy them, so they sit in liquid nitrogen indefinitely. Recent estimates show there are approximately 400,000 frozen embryos in IVF clinics across the country.

The ability to freeze eggs would help to alleviate this predicament. Many women feel less attached to eggs than embryos, so freezing them, and eventually discarding them would present little, if any, moral discomfort. However, there are major steps to overcome in order for egg freezing to become a viable option on a wide scale. Unlike individual sperm cells, and tiny three- or five-day-old embryos, a human egg is more like one big, bulging, delicate, water balloon. Therefore attempts to freeze eggs using contemporary methods for sperm and embryos result in damage beyond repair. All the water, plus the monstrous size of a mature egg, mean ice crystals form and can destroy the fragile structures inside. Despite the quandary, freezing the raw materials of reproduction, including eggs, is currently available, and is poised to help launch the next women's reproductive revolution.

Eggs-tending Your Biological Clock

One company is well on its way to offering egg freezing to the masses. Extend Fertility, Inc., was launched with the sole purpose of providing an egg freezing service to women who would like to preserve their biological clocks well beyond nature's timetable. Extend Fertility's 30-something founder and CEO, Christy Jones, was her company's first customer. "There is a tremendous need out there for women to have this kind of insurance policy. The number of single women in their 30s has tripled since 1970, and now stands at 30 percent of all women. And today, one in five women waits until 35 or older to start her family. These are the women who hear their biological clocks clanging, and have no way to stop it. Now they will." Jones is quick to point out that this kind of insurance is not guaranteed. "We offer information without playing to women's fears. We are factual with the limited scientific data and the current success rates, so women can make their own informed decision. It's not a 100 percent insurance policy, but it does at least expand a woman's options."

Another company, ViaCell, Inc., has licensed and is supporting clinical trials at Boston IVF on a new technique for egg freezing, with the hopes of offering it to the public sometime in the next two years. Several independent reproductive medicine clinics are also now offering the service. Most experts put the number of actual babies born from frozen eggs at somewhere between 100 and 200 worldwide. So the various techniques do work; however, even the best success rates are of limited value given the relatively few children born thus far.

The Slow Freezing Technique

This is the most traditional technique employed for freezing eggs; it has also been studied and tweaked by more scientists and embryologists than any other. It is the basic method used by several clinics around the country, as well as those affiliated with Extend Fertility. A group of investigators in Italy first revealed *slowly* freezing eggs that have been submerged in a kind of antifreeze or cryoprotectant could actually work with acceptable success rates. (Note: In the medical literature, eggs are always referred to as *oocytes* and the process of freezing is known as *cryopreservation*.) These researchers showed that when eggs are exposed to a cryoprotectant along with a type of simple sugar called sucrose for up to 15 minutes, then slowly frozen, a high rate of survival after thawing (82 percent) resulted compared to other methods.

The antifreeze helps protect the eggs from crystal formation because it seeps inside the egg and displaces some of the water; the sucrose facilitates this dehydration process, because it acts like a sump pump by sitting outside the egg, drawing water out, thereby further reducing the possibility of crystals. With this technique, the sucrose surrounds the egg cell and extracts the water via osmosis. Once this is accomplished, the eggs become dehydrated; they are smaller and more compact—sort of vacuum-packed—in preparation for freezing.

Recently, three U.S. clinics have advanced this method to the point of good survival, fertilization, pregnancy, and birth rates. Jeffrey Boldt, Ph.D., scientific and program director at Assisted Fertility Services in Indianapolis, was the first to publish a scientific paper with data on pregnancy and birth rates. His freezing technique yielded a 74-percent survival rate, a 59-percent fertilization rate, and five babies, including one set of twins. Boldt started with just 15 women using

162

this protocol, making his take-home baby rate 26.6 percent, which is comparable to the rate for frozen embryos. His work has continued, and his most recent data brings his pregnancy rate to 34.3 percent—better than the latest CDC averages for frozen embryos. He's optimistic about his work. "It's coming along—all the kids are doing great as near as I can tell."

Embryologist Barry Behr, Ph.D., HCLD, director of IVF/ART Laboratories at Stanford, has been working on advancing this technique as well. "I'm able to demonstrate that the results are very repeatable and that we should expect the survival rates of these frozen eggs [to be] between 60 and 80 percent, with fertilization rates around 70 percent. If it looks good after thawing, we know from experience, it's going to work."

A Jacksonville, Florida, clinic has also had success with the slow freezing method, and is offering it to women undergoing treatment, as well as those who want to preserve their eggs. The Florida Institute for Reproductive Medicine has reported pregnancy rates at 28.4 percent with data showing on average it takes 19 eggs to produce a baby, with that average dropping to just 12 for women who freeze their eggs while they are still fertile.

So women can expect a possible 20- to 30-percent viable pregnancy rate using this method. These are far better odds than women face once their clocks strike midnight. On average, a 40-year-old woman's chances of having a baby using her own fresh eggs, is around 10 percent, and after that, even less. Behr points out, "Remember, you're dealing with whatever the odds are of thawing these eggs out, five to 10 years from now. They could be higher. But even if they remain between 20 and 30 percent—that's versus the chances of getting pregnant at 42 or 44, when we're talking just 3 to 5 percent. I think it's really going to change many of the options that women have with respect to building families, and careers."

The "Sweeter the Better" Method

Boston researchers and entrepreneurs are banking on a variation of the slow freeze technique. Thomas Toth, M.D., of Massachusetts General Hospital, developed the method (Harvard Medical School, ViaCell, Inc., and Boston IVF are also involved in current work) using a cryoprotectant sugar called trehalose. Rather than depending on osmosis to remove water from the egg, Toth is injecting the special sugar compound right into the cell with recent reported survival rates of over 60 percent. It is believed the trehalose naturally protects cells because this substance is found in many organisms living in harsh environments. These animals survive extreme conditions including dehydration, desiccation, and freezing. Toth has been studying what happens to animals, such as salamanders, when a deep freeze sets in. "They appear to go into a state of suspended animation, and they accumulate these sugars inside their cells which allow them to develop into this very stable state." He says that if he can mimic this effect in human eggs, it may provide a more successful method of freezing them. "Our hope is that the benefits of sugar will provide a more natural effect, and it could be an improvement over current technologies."

Turning Eggs to Glass

Another approach called *vitrification* is based on the idea that rather than allowing any ice crystals to form, they would be totally eliminated, creating a glassy-like suspended animation of the cell. During this procedure, extremely high levels of cryoprotectants (antifreeze) penetrate the cell, completely purging it of water. The eggs are then quickly dropped into a deep freeze, instantly shutting down all biological activity. Vitrification takes about 10 minutes; whereas the slow freeze method can take much longer.

The advantage of vitrification is that it's quick, but the embryologist has to work rapidly and accurately, because the concentrations of cryoprotectants are so high that any extended exposure could completely destroy the cell. A few groups of researchers are working on maximizing the vitrification solutions and timing the process.

One group in Seoul, Korea, has published a study showing six successful pregnancies following freezing and thawing of eggs using this method. The results yielded a pregnancy rate of 21.4 percent, that's six pregnancies out of 28 transfers. This rate is similar to those achieved with slow cooling, but like many other studies of this nature, the number of women participating was small, underscoring the need for further research.

Another group has achieved an egg cell survival rate of 81 to 85 percent following vitrification of more than a thousand human eggs.

It took just 11.5 minutes to freeze them and 15 minutes to warm them, compared to the slow freeze—rapid thaw method needing 90 minutes to freeze and about 30 minutes to thaw. This group recently fertilized 13 previously vitrified human eggs, and four resulting embryos were transferred, but no pregnancy resulted. Five of the healthiest extra embryos have been re-vitrified, and may be used to try again. One of the researchers, Juergen Liebermann, Ph.D., of the Fertility Center of Illinois, is confident the effort will eventually produce viable pregnancies. "This is a very promising case, and we will continue to move forward with this clinical work."

Sunny Side up or Hard-Boiled?

It may seem hard to believe, but there is an ongoing debate whether freezing eggs is a good idea. Some experts believe it gives women a false sense of security because the success rates are still relatively low. However, others have ethical concerns about providing a medical service for social goals. Robert Stillman, M.D., medical director of the Shady Grove Fertility Center outside Washington, D.C., argues, "I think medicine is for treating patients who have a medical disorder. I had a woman who said, 'I want a gestational surrogate because I don't want stretch marks." I had another who said, 'I am a busy lawyer, my clients will suffer, so I want a gestational surrogate.' Those are social goals. Freezing eggs for a woman who is about to have her ovaries removed or go through radiation therapy for cancer is one thing. But to do it just to hang out longer or advance a career may be very laudable from a social standpoint, but isn't the role, I believe, of medicine."

Of course there is a chorus of others who stand firmly on the other side of the fence. "I disagree," says Richard Paulson, M.D., chief of the division of Reproductive Endocrinology and Infertility at the University of Southern California School of Medicine. "I think that is totally what medicine is about. To me, we don't have enough respect for gametes. Gametes die all the time. A woman that has two children, has two eggs that successfully fertilized, the other 2 million are all dead someplace. And how many billions and billions of sperm die every day everywhere? So I think to store them is perfectly reasonable." Embryologist Barry Behr, Ph.D., maintains anyone who has a problem with advancing egg freezing "sees the glass as half empty—because this is going to be the biggest advance in our field this decade, no question. Having this option for women is huge."

165

Others who favor advancing the science of egg freezing are those who are morally uncomfortable with the idea of freezing embryos for indefinite storage. Many believe, if egg freezing can eventually yield similar success rates as frozen embryos for IVF patients, there would be no need to fertilize so many leftover eggs, only to store the resulting embryos with no clear plan for their use or disposal. Those uneasy with the idea of frozen embryos, for either religious or other reasons, would likely prefer to store their eggs.

Another, more futuristic, argument for advancing this technology would be to develop donor egg banks, much like donor sperm banks. Some observers contend, if eggs can be frozen and stored with similar success rates as frozen sperm, it would eliminate the dicey business of finding and paying individual egg donors. The process and fees could then be standardized, with couples choosing an egg donor at a storage depot rather than through an agency, over the Internet, or in a local paper.

Other Eggs-tension Research

In order to retrieve individual mature eggs for freezing, a woman must undergo the same ovarian stimulation regimen as she would for a standard IVF procedure. This requires at least two weeks in a rushed case, to over a month, before eggs can be retrieved. It is time consuming, especially for cancer patients who often must begin their chemotherapy or radiation treatment promptly. Because of these potential obstacles, doctors have experimented with removing ovarian tissue, and even whole ovaries, to preserve fertility. The idea is to freeze it—that is, suspend it in time—and transplant it back to the body, perhaps years later.

Recently, researchers from Brussels, Belgium, announced a potential breakthrough that could mark a major step forward in *ovarian tissue transplantation*—the first pregnancy and birth in a woman after having her tissue transplanted back. Before undergoing chemotherapy for advanced Hodgkin's lymphoma in 1997, the now 32-year-old woman had some of her ovarian tissue removed and frozen, and doctors left one ovary inside her body. The tissue was transplanted back just below her existing ovary, and four months later she began to ovulate. Doctors say her baby was conceived naturally, but they can't say for certain whether the egg that was fertilized came from the transplanted tissue or her ovary, which somehow could have begun working again.

Kutluk Oktay, M.D., of the Center for Reproductive Medicine and Infertility at the Weill Medical College, Cornell University, has pioneered techniques for ovarian tissue transplantation. His work, however, has focused on combining ovarian tissue transplantation with IVF. Just a few months prior to this latest development, Oktay and colleagues announced they had produced the first viable human embryo using this method.

In Oktay's case the 30-year-old woman had one ovary removed, then underwent chemotherapy, and was soon confirmed to be in menopause—her ovarian tissue wasn't transplanted back until six years later. Rather than next to her existing ovary, Oktay implanted 15 tissue grafts underneath the skin of the patient's abdomen. After three months, the patient felt a pea-sized lump—a follicle had formed. No question, the ovarian tissue had begun to function again. Researchers even checked her remaining intact ovary and found no follicle development, so they were sure the transplanted strips had kickstarted her biological clock again: her estrogen levels increased; her FSH dropped; and she started producing follicles. Her menopause had reversed.

Oktay retrieved 20 eggs from beneath her skin; two fertilized, one embryo stopped growing at three cells, the other grew to four cells and was transferred to the patient's uterus. No pregnancy developed; though it is clear from this study that it is possible to create human embryos in vitro using this type of ovarian tissue preservation.

Scientific breakthroughs take time, and Oktay says we must have patience. "We're dealing with just one patient, so I think it's normal to have slow progress or repeated failures in the beginning. It's just a matter of trying enough times and figuring out what's right, what's not. But each time we do it, we learn something else and it makes the next procedure better." Oktay admits that at first they weren't even able to handle the eggs without damaging them. "If you collect them too late, the eggs are old, if you collect them too soon, they're too young. You can't use the same criteria you use with ovaries in a normal location. It's like reinventing IVF all over again."

Researchers are confident because the procedure has produced baby mice, sheep, and most recently, a monkey, so it should be able to produce human babies too. Because the reported human pregnancy was naturally conceived rather than due to IVF, it remains to be seen if scientists can confirm whether the transplanted ovarian tissue produced the baby.

Limited study has been conducted on removing entire ovaries for storage and future use. Though researchers have successfully frozen entire ovaries, it appears doing so is more challenging than freezing ovarian tissue strips. If the technique could be improved, it would theoretically provide more tissue, and therefore more eggs to use in the future. However, there are many who question the idea of removing a whole healthy ovary as a hedge against future reproductive decline—even in the case of cancer patients—because the science thus far simply does not support the idea.

Pros and Cons of Ovarian Tissue Preservation

The most convincing reason to continue this research is that it eliminates the need to use fertility drugs to stimulate egg production. Imagine—no daily shots! This would be ideal for some cancer patients; it may also be more desirable for others who would like to preserve their fertility. Extracting ovarian tissue would require perhaps a three-day procedure, including minor laparoscopic (keyhole) surgery from start to finish, as opposed to several weeks of injecting fertility drugs and many appointments for monitoring before undergoing egg retrieval, a minor surgical procedure.

In addition, because it eliminates the need for *mature* eggs, this procedure could be available to much younger women, even prepubescent girls, who risk losing their fertility at a very young age due to treatments that wreak havoc on eggs. Other advantages include the ease of freezing these smaller primordial eggs; and the availability of more eggs, because hundreds, if not thousands, would be frozen rather than just a dozen or two.

The main drawback at the moment? The technique is new, and unproven in people. Several clinics are offering ovarian tissue freezing to cancer patients, but there is a tremendous amount of work to do before it can be used on a greater scale. Aside from confirming the origin of the egg that resulted in this recent birth, researchers are working on several other issues: the optimal freezing and thawing technique, because many eggs in the tissue strips still die in the process; and the best time for egg retrieval from the transplant site. Plus, this method of potential fertility preservation may not be appropriate for older patients because it relies on large numbers of healthy eggs. A woman over 30 may not have enough; and if too much ovarian tissue is removed, a younger woman may end up entering menopause sooner, defeating the purpose of fertility preservation, giving her *less* time to conceive naturally.

Growing Eggs Somewhere Else

Mice as egg factories?

What if there was no need to transplant the tissue back into the woman's body to grow and mature the eggs? What if embryologists could thaw out the frozen strips and put them in a type of incubator along with the properly timed hormonal triggers that would awaken primordial follicles, energize them, and induce them to mature to the point that they would be ready for fertilization? The answer is: that would change everything!

Such a scenario, if perfected, would totally eliminate the need for all those injections to stimulate ovaries to produce lots of *mature* eggs prior to IVF; all you would need is a biopsy to obtain a small amount of ovarian tissue that you could freeze, and years later instruct the clinic to grow, fertilize, and produce embryos so you could start your family whenever you would like. A couple of years later you could call back and ask them to start the process again for your next child. Though scientists are working toward this goal, they aren't quite there yet. In fact, they are a long way from being able to take human ovarian tissue full of tiny primordial follicles (containing your most immature eggs), and grow them in a laboratory. Although they have had some success with eggs that are *almost* mature—more on this momentarily.

One place scientists have been able to grow these very early follicles is in other animals! Several groups have transplanted human ovarian tissue into mice, which have been genetically bred without an immune system, so they can't reject the foreign tissue. Amazingly, ovarian grafts growing in mice have consistently produced potentially viable human eggs.

Other groups have also experimented with transplanting ovarian tissue from a variety of animals into mice and other species. Researchers at Purdue University and a fertility clinic in Indianapolis even tried incubating previously frozen elephant ovarian tissue in mice. They succeeded, and produced one elephant egg—in a mouse! Recently, researchers in Australia took another leap forward with xenotransplantation (across species) and grew wallaby eggs in mice and rats. They transferred the embryos to surrogate wallaby mothers, but so far there are no wallaby babies. This cross-species incubation technique has, however, produced baby mice following growing mouse ovarian tissue in rats, retrieving the eggs, fertilizing them, and transferring the embryos back into surrogate mouse mothers.

Success with such reproductive technology has obvious implications for the protection of endangered species, but some experts say it could prove a major advance for people too. Cancer patients, in particular, usually can't undergo ovarian stimulation with fertility drugs, and transplanting their own ovarian tissue grafts may not be advisable because the tissue could contain cancer cells. Using animals as hosts would eliminate the risk of the cancer recurring. Even a woman's ovarian tissue that is known to carry cancer could theoretically be transplanted to a mouse with her *healthy* eggs produced and removed for fertilization and transfer back to her uterus, or perhaps to a gestational carrier. In addition, mice could be used for those who would rather not undergo the minor surgery to transplant the tissue back; the stimulating drugs; and the egg retrieval necessary to obtain matured eggs from the growing follicles. However, aside from the "yuck" factor, concerns remain about disease transmission from mice to women via the eggs, and whether egg incubation in a different species would somehow affect normal development in subsequent offspring.

In Vitro Maturation

Many who look into the reproductive medicine crystal ball think using animals as egg manufacturers would only be an interim step. That's because the hypothetical laboratory-based primordial egg incubator idea is not all that far-fetched. The fact is, it has been done in mice. Scientists in one experiment used *newborn* mouse ovarian tissue, so the primordial eggs were as far from the maturation process as possible. Taking their best guess at mixing a concoction to mimic the environment that would trigger egg growth and keep them developing, scientists produced mature mouse eggs without ever putting them back into any living animal. The eggs then fertilized, and the embryos

170

were placed into surrogate mouse mothers. The pregnancy rate was extremely low; out of 190 transferred embryos, only two mice were born. Nevertheless, researchers took the eggs from newborns, and matured them in vitro all the way to fertilization, producing live offspring.

One day, research may reveal the precise mechanism that selects a set of primordial human follicles and rouses them to come out of their comatose state and begin the long run toward the maturation finish line. Scientists are trying to unravel what hormonal and molecular switches are critical to triggering the initial stages of follicle and egg development, as well as the signaling mechanisms that keep the process going. What they know is there is a tremendous amount of communication going on between the egg and the cells contained within the follicle, and between the follicle and the rest of the hormonal system. Once this complicated cell-to-cell-to-body messaging network is revealed, scientists can start trying to duplicate it in the laboratory.

Although it will likely be some time before embryologists can incubate early human primordial follicles in their labs, researchers can now retrieve *immature* eggs from women, induce them to fully mature in a petri dish, fertilize them, and produce healthy babies. The latest published reports indicate that approximately 300 babies have been born through the use of this special laboratory culturing technique, also known as in vitro maturation (IVM).

These human eggs are cultured for the very last part of the maturation process, a course that is thought to begin in the ovary anywhere from three to six months before an egg is ready to be ovulated. In most of these studies, eggs that were partially mature were taken and induced to finish the process in the laboratory for the last 24 to 48 hours. Much of the success has been with women who have polycystic ovarian syndrome (PCOS), a condition where women produce lots of immature eggs, but can still be infertile. These women also run a very high risk of ovarian hyperstimulation syndrome (OHSS), a dangerous and potentially life-threatening condition if they undergo treatment with fertility drugs.

In these women, retrieving antral (immature) follicles and maturing them in the laboratory can lead to take-home babies. But a couple of clinics have suggested and tried IVM for older women or poor responders who are resistant to ovarian stimulation protocols for IVF.

These women's follicles often grow slowly, and sometimes few, if any, become fully mature. Still, poor responders generally do produce a good amount of *almost* mature follicles. Unfortunately, without the standard four to 12 large *mature* follicles, REs usually cancel these cycles due to poor response. But those who are believers in IVM say retrieving all follicles, including the small ones, and finishing the maturation process in the laboratory, can offer a much greater chance of pregnancy. Pregnancies and births have been reported in poor responders whose doctors decided to retrieve their immature eggs and culture them in vitro rather than cancel the cycle altogether.

These successes have inspired further investigation into using IVM in natural cycles, that is, without prior ovarian stimulation with fertility drugs. The ovaries produce upwards of 20 follicles each month, of which generally only one will become fully matured, and will be ovulated. Even women with slowing clocks produce some follicles each month. So why not skip the drugs, retrieve the less developed eggs, and simply mature them in the lab? Many believe, with continued advances in IVM, this technique will become routine.

In addition, if you combine the possibility of freezing immature eggs or ovarian tissue that can be grown for a short while in a mouse, then matured completely in the lab, this could usher in yet another wave of options for women. Some observers see a day when women undergoing C-sections or other abdominal surgery will have some ovarian tissue removed at the same time to donate to an egg bank, with the option of using it at a later date. Others believe that obtaining ovarian tissue from a biopsy, freezing and thawing it, then using IVM to prepare for fertilization will be more attractive, more effective, and less expensive than going through a stimulated cycle with fertility drugs. Some day, women will have these choices available to them.

Recipes for Making or Improving Eggs and Sperm

Can two moms make it right?

The headline reads, "Scientists Create Mouse with Two Moms." That's right, no sperm necessary. Following the report in the journal *Nature*, it is clear that eggs can be genetically manipulated so that they mimic sperm. The result in this unprecedented investigation: a single mouse that carries the DNA from *two* female mice; this offspring went on to mature and reproduce the normal way.

But don't toss your boyfriend or husband just yet. Though it worked in mice, that doesn't mean it could ever happen, at least not with this method, in humans. Here, researchers were able to genetically engineer mice, which essentially produced DNA that acted as if it came from sperm rather than an egg. The genetic switches they identified, and turned off, are called *imprints*. Manipulating these imprints won't change the genetic inheritance, it simply either turns genes on or off, because only one switch in each gene pair can be on at any one time. So if it's *on* in the female gene, it has to be *off* in the male gene. In this case, scientists were able to produce a mouse whose normally imprinted "on" female gene was turned off, so that it could trick the egg into thinking it came from a sperm. Interestingly, there are about 90 imprinted genes in mice, but scientists only had to manipulate one. They believe this one adjustment may have started a cascade of events that transformed the others into paternal rather than maternal imprints.

Even in mice, success was no easy feat. Dr. Tomoiro Kono and his team at the Tokyo University of Agriculture produced 457 eggs that combined the two mothers' genetic material, and *two* babies were born—only one survived to adulthood. That's less than a 1-percent success rate, and nobody is sure if the mouse is completely normal. Still, such a breakthrough is sure to spur further research along this route, and who knows, perhaps one day, 30-something women who haven't met Mr. Right, may not need to....

Body Cells to Make Egg Cells

Another possibility on the horizon for the clock that's on its last tock: creating artificial eggs out of the DNA from a woman's own *somatic* cells, or body cells. By using the woman's DNA, she can produce her own genetically related child. Researchers have created artificial eggs capable of fertilization first in mice, and then in humans. At this point, though, the technique remains highly experimental, and somewhat controversial.

Researchers remove the nucleus from a donor egg and then insert the nucleus of the intended mother's somatic cell into that egg. Next, they use a jolt of electricity to induce the new cell to split its full compliment of 46 chromosomes down to 23, a process called *haploidization*. Because the egg has only half the required number of chromosomes, it can now be fertilized with the father's sperm. Hence, half of the resulting embryo's genes will come from its mother, and half from its father.

Unlike the genes in the mother's natural eggs, which have been shuffled into unique combinations (refer to *chiasmata* in Chapter 2) of her mother and father's genes, in this case, the mother's half will be an exact duplicate of her own genes. Gianpiero Palermo, M.D., of the Center for Reproductive Medicine and Infertility at the Weill Medical College of Cornell University in New York City, developed the technique. He is confident it can provide a way for a woman with poor egg quality due to premature menopause, or natural age-related fertility decline, to have her own genetic child rather than using eggs and genetics donated from another woman. "This would help women of any age. I don't think it matters if the egg is identical to the mother, that's fine. You still need the sperm to complete the process, so you would have a unique individual that belongs to the couple."

Palermo is passionate about finding ways for reproductively older women to have children; he insists it's where this area of medical research is heading, "In our field, we have solved tubal problems with IVF, we've solved male issues with ICSI, now we are bumping against the wall, and the wall is age-related infertility."

Cytoplasmic and Nuclear Transfer

These techniques apply the same principle as Palermo's work with somatic cells, except they rely on the DNA contained inside a woman's natural *eggs* rather than body cells. The key ingredient is donated egg cell *cytoplasm*. The cytoplasm is comprised of all the fluid and structures called organelles inside the egg that surround the nucleus. It is believed, and there is evidence to show, that certain organelles, called *mitochondria*, provide the fuel to power the egg's activities, including the all-important maturation process, fertilization, and early embryonic development. Without a sufficient number of energized mitochondria, which contain their own DNA to orchestrate their many tasks, it is believed an egg will be unable to perform all the precise strenuous steps necessary to prepare for fertilization and continue to develop once fertilization begins.

One study shows there are many more mutations in the mitochondria of older eggs than those of younger ones. In subjects between the ages of 26 and 36 researchers found a mutation in one egg out of 11 patients, but in patients between the ages of 37 and 42, they found 17 mutations in 10 patients. That's a difference in mitochondrial mutation rate of 4.4 percent in younger patients, compared to 39.5 percent in the older patients. Researchers believe these mutations, and possibly other cytoplasmic factors, affect the quality of eggs in older patients. They hypothesize that pumping older, more lethargic eggs with a small dose of younger cytoplasm from a donor egg may be all that is necessary to reenergize them, so the older eggs can produce a viable pregnancy.

Some preliminary research reveals they may be right. In the late 1990s researchers at the Institute for Reproductive Medicine and Science of Saint Barnabas in New Jersey injected the eggs of patients with donor cytoplasm and achieved several pregnancies in women who had failed previous IVF treatments. In all, 12 out of 28 cases produced a pregnancy and 15 healthy children were born. In another, more recent investigation conducted in China, researchers collected two mature eggs from a 46-year-old patient, then isolated thousands of mitochondria from some of the patient's other reproductive cells. They injected about 3,000 mitochondria into each egg, and both fertilized. One went on to develop normally, and after transfer, the woman became pregnant. Unfortunately, the pregnancy ended in miscarriage in the ninth week. However, the case was published because it was believed to represent the *oldest* woman to have ART and achieve a pregnancy with her *own* eggs—in all of China.

Because cytoplasmic transfer using donor eggs has come under scrutiny by the Food and Drug Administration (more on this later), one clinic has begun injecting a patient's eggs with a small amount of cytoplasm from one of her own eggs, which is essentially sacrificed, rather than use the cytoplasm from another woman's donor egg. Dr. Michael Fakih, of the Fakih Institute of Reproductive Sciences and Technology just outside Detroit, calls the procedure *self-cytoplasmic transfer*. He says so long as a woman produces a few mature eggs, even though she's a poor responder, he can use the cytoplasm from one egg to boost the rest of them. He's only performed this technique on a handful of patients, some that have been refused treatment at other clinics because they insist on using their own eggs rather than donor eggs. Fakih says so far most have achieved pregnancy. "We are very excited about this. I'm a true believer. All these patients have failed IVF before, and with their own cytoplasm they got pregnant. So it's clearly telling us something."

Nuclear transfer is a variation on this theme. The difference is that rather than removing donor or self-cytoplasm and injecting it into the patient's eggs, researchers take the nucleus out of the intended mother's egg and transfer it into a donor egg that has had its nucleus removed, but is still full of cytoplasm. The result is the patient retains all of her genes within her nuclear DNA, while at the same time the nucleus derives all the benefit from the donor's cytoplasm. This technique has been shown to be promising in mice and in limited preliminary research in humans.

The doctor who pioneered this type of "nuclear transfer" received institutional review board approval for the first human study back in 1997. James Grifo, M.D., Ph.D., director of the Program for In Vitro Fertilization, Reproductive Surgery, and Infertility at the New York University School of Medicine, reported the results at a scientific meeting the following year. Essentially, he and his team were able to take eggs from five patients, remove the germinal vesicles (nuclei containing 46 chromosomes prior to meiosis), and put them into donor eggs that had their nuclei removed. They electrically activated the eggs, fertilized them, and created embryos that were chromosomally normal. Within days after this research was reported and it made the front pages of newspapers including the *Washington Post*, the federal government instructed Grifo to halt his research.

The U.S. Food and Drug Administration said it had jurisdiction over his research because it involved cloning technology, and required that he submit an investigational new drug application in order to be considered for approval. Grifo insists he is not creating a new drug, nor is his goal at all related to cloning. He argues he is conducting medical research in a nonprofit academic institution that should be regulated through the traditional route—institutional review board approval and patients' informed consent—not governmental control. He says this unprecedented restriction is impeding progress for patients. "We can correct the eggs of older women and help them have babies, or we can even use this for patients who have mitochondrial disease so they don't pass on disorders to their children, but we can't, because the government won't let us."

176

Grifo is not alone. The FDA placed the same restrictions on cytoplasmic transfer techniques as well. Grifo feels strongly that both cytoplasmic and nuclear transfer research should be allowed to continue. Recently, he consulted with researchers in China—where the regulations were more lenient. They identified a patient who failed to produce any viable embryos, but using the nuclear transfer technique, produced several. Doctors transferred four to her uterus, and a triplet pregnancy resulted. The couple, and doctors, decided to reduce the pregnancy to twins. Unfortunately, four months later, the amniotic sac containing one of the fetuses broke, the baby was born prematurely and died soon after. Because that delivery opened the birth canal, it left the other fetus vulnerable to infection. Despite giving the patient antibiotics, a silent infection resulted, and the last baby's umbilical cord failed. This baby delivered prematurely and also died.

The tragic outcome caused an uproar in the mainstream U.S. media. Grifo agrees this case is heart wrenching, but he says it only had a tragic ending because of poor obstetrical care. He adds that testing on the fetuses showed they were all normal. "What happened had nothing to do with the technique, it had to do with the multiple gestation. In retrospect, we shouldn't have put back four embryos, but we never thought it would work three out of four times. It's a shame the work had to be done in China, rather than here," he adds. Just days before the Chinese team and Grifo reported this study at a scientific meeting in 2003, China announced sweeping new regulations prohibiting human cloning and placing strict controls on fertility research, including nuclear transfer.

It appears for now, both nuclear transfer and cytoplasmic transfer remain on indefinite hold.

Stem Cells:
The Seeds to Grow Eggs and Sperm

Adult Ovarian Stem Cells...a New Possibility

Certainly one of the most exciting developments in reproductive medicine has been the recent discovery of evidence that ovarian stem cells appear to be producing *new* eggs in *adult* mice. The finding shatters the basic tenet in reproductive medicine that female mammals are born with all the eggs they will ever have. This has tremendous implications for future research; among the most pressing is the identification of similar stem cell evidence and new egg production in humans. If the same is found to be true in women's ovaries, it is easy to envision a day when a simple ovarian biopsy during the most fertile years—early 20s—would secure enough egg-producing stem cells to freeze them for later use. Lead author of the study, Jonathan Tilly, Ph.D., of Massachusetts General Hospital, is excited about the prospects. "If they do exist, we can harvest them, even just small numbers of them, and expand them in the dish, just make more of them pharmacologically, and then we could freeze some away, and also put them right back in the ovary, and essentially regrow ovaries."

Stem cells have been shown to freeze well, so it wouldn't matter how many actual eggs the biopsy contained, because you could simply thaw the stem cells 10, 20, 30 years later and make more stem cells or as many eggs as needed, then return the extra stem cells to the deep freeze. The rejuvenated stem cells could then produce eggs in the ovary for natural conception, or they could be produced, matured, and fertilized in vitro, and the resulting embryos could be transferred into the mother's uterus. These procedures would provide the same chances of a healthy pregnancy as a 20-something-year-old, and the process could be repeated whenever the woman would like to have another child.

Tilly says this scenario is not science fiction. He believes it's highly likely they will find a similar mechanism at work in human ovaries, and once they do, "there's absolutely no reason that adult stem cell-based technologies can not be developed for manipulating ovarian function. Absolutely no reason."

According to published reports, Tilly's team has already accomplished this in mice. Researchers have isolated egg-producing stem cells, and have discovered a gene that seems to regulate them. When the gene is knocked out, or shut down, the mice produce more eggs. They have also developed a molecule that appears to affect egg production. When injected into mice just prior to puberty, the mice produce almost twice as many eggs as they normally do. All of these developments, if applicable to women, bode well for prolonging biological clocks. "The future looks bright," says Tilly.

Women might maintain their fertility well into old age, if they choose to do so. In addition to reversing age-related infertility, such a

178

breakthrough would have tremendous potential implications for women's health given that the same technology would allow women to stave off menopause, perhaps for good. The big question is whether delaying the menopause would also postpone all the health-related consequences that generally follow. Given that hormone replacement therapy proved largely a failure in postmenopausal women, perhaps keeping the ovaries functioning longer, producing natural hormones, and keeping the clock ticking, could prevent many of the health risks tied to menopause.

"If we get a good handle on the mechanism, there's absolutely no reason to think that we couldn't jumpstart these cells, if they were getting old, or alternatively keep them from dying.... That's what we've been working on for the past 10 years. So the same technology could very easily be applied to these cells, if that is the mechanism of aging," according to Tilly.

Embryonic Stem Cells

This avenue of research has overthrown yet another previously held scientific belief: that it is impossible to create eggs or sperm out of embryonic stem cells. New research has shown both are indeed possible. A collaboration of scientists from several research institutions in Boston, including the Whitehead Institute for Biomedical Research, Massachusetts General Hospital, Harvard Medical School, and Children's Hospital Boston, isolated stem cells from mouse embryos, cultured them in vitro, and induced them to become primordial germ cells; researchers then allowed them to continue to develop and found they became functional sperm. Though they lacked tails, when researchers injected them into eggs, they were capable of fertilization. These stem cell–derived sperm-created embryos with a full complement of chromosomes. It remains to be seen whether further experimentation will produce normal embryonic development, and the true test of success: normal baby mice.

Eggs from stem cells? Yes, that's now possible too. Scientists at the School of Veterinary Medicine and the Center for Research on Reproduction and Women's Health at the University of Pennsylvania isolated stem cells from embryos and coaxed them into developing into egg-like cells. Though some structures appeared swollen, most looked remarkably like typical eggs given they were the proper size

179

and enclosed in a shell that appeared to function like the outer coating in a normal egg cell. These eggs were then released from the cells surrounding them and appeared to mature. However, rather than suspending development until fertilization, these eggs spontaneously divided, becoming embryos on their own. Their developmental potential remains unknown.

Being able to create stem cells, and then instruct them to become what ever cell is desired, could allow researchers to develop new cellular treatments for a multitude of diseases, including infertility. The ability to manufacture stem cells from adult cells would mean researchers could grow unlimited numbers of stem cells for research and at the same time eliminate the ethical dilemma of using human embryos for such research. Using body cells to create eggs that spontaneously produce embryos and then harvest stem cells may hold the key to individualized medical treatment, where therapeutic tissues could be customized and returned to the same person without any problems with tissue rejection. For example, such tissues could be developed to halt cancer or create brand-new eggs for a woman who wishes to have her own genetic child. Sounds futuristic, but most scientists agree that with continued research, these advances are possible.

Cloning

Notice I haven't used the "C" word until now. That's because whenever you use the word *cloning*, it makes the ground tremble beneath just about everyone. So it's no surprise it is often invoked in mainstream TV, newspaper headlines, and stories pertaining to many of the topics already discussed—the "C" word sells. The bottom line is that you can't do any of the research involving eggs, sperm, stem cells, or any combination thereof, without using some of the *techniques* involved in cloning. As soon as researchers take a nucleus out of one cell and put it into another, or combine genetic materials from different sources, they are using cloning methods. However, that doesn't mean that what is happening is cloning, or that the goal is to make an exact copy of anyone. On the contrary, once fertilization takes place—the addition of a separate, and unique complement of chromosomes—the notion of an exact duplicate is out the window. Therefore, using a cloning technique does not de facto result in a clone.

However, the opposite can be true; you don't necessarily have to use cloning techniques to get a "clone." For instance, the eggs that were created at the University of Pennsylvania simply grew from stem cells, and then "spontaneously" developed into embryos—they were, in fact, embryo "clones" of the mouse whose nuclear DNA was used, because the eggs were never fertilized with sperm.

I present this distinction because it is important to separate *real* cloning from the research that is often misrepresented as cloning. What the Ralians tried to fool us into thinking they were doing was real human cloning, making an exact duplicate of a person. Dolly the sheep and countless other animals have been cloned. Some people reason that human cloning should be pursued as a treatment for infertility, because nature produces clones all the time, as in the case of identical twins. Others cringe at the idea that a person would want to clone him- or herself; that is, create a child that, in the case of a woman, would be both her younger identical twin and her daughter. If the scientific evidence weren't so dismal when it comes to real cloning, the topic might be more of a pressing issue. Yes, more than likely, it is possible to clone a human being, but all the animal investigations so far show it is extremely difficult to do so, and the animal clones simply do not live a full life span.

The reason scientists believe this occurs is (and this is a very simplified explanation) when you produce a creature from a single *adult* somatic cell, that cell has already used up about half of its dividing capacity, so using it to start another life all over again, only gives the offspring what the original cell had left to go—about half a life. This predetermined number of cell divisions in a cell is called the Hayflick Limit. Why would you want risk imposing this kind of limit on your child—just so you could see your green eyes or curly brown hair in a younger version? It makes no sense; it seems unfair, and cruel.

Using *techniques* that manipulate eggs, sperm, and stem cells, with other goals in mind, however, is another story. So long as we are not talking about stamping out exact copies of people, and we are only interested in alleviating suffering, whether it's due to a catatonic biological clock or life-threatening disease, there's no question such research using cloning *techniques* ought to continue.

Threats to Progress

Many Americans see all attempts at manipulating reproductive cells, especially those that have fused to become embryos, no matter how this is accomplished, as unethical, possibly immoral, or at the very least dangerous. They believe a seven- or eight-cell embryo is the same as a 5-year-old romping through a playground or even the living equivalent to a surgeon repairing his fourth heart for the week. The reasoning extends to all embryos, even if they are cloned from body cells with the intention of harvesting stem cells, not reproduction; and this camp steadfastly maintains that these so-called innocent *lives* cannot be manipulated nor destroyed for any reason. Sounds like the abortion debate, except here the discussion is about something microscopic, consisting of eight or so cells, that cannot feel, think, laugh, cry, or contribute to society in any way.

This point of view has stymied research since President George W. Bush's decision to halt federal funding for stem cell research that uses any source of stem cells other than those already created. However, Bush's decision simply slowed an already limping pace of research requiring human embryos. Currently, there is little federal funding for studies on anything IVF-related, and virtually none for scientific endeavors that necessitate the use of human embryos. Much of this investigation is privately funded, with no change in sight.

In addition, in 2001 the FDA stepped into the reproductive medicine arena. Several clinics received personal letters prohibiting scientists from continuing either cytoplasmic transfer from donor eggs, or nuclear transfer into donor eggs. It informed scientists and institutional review boards that the FDA has complete jurisdiction over this area of research, and anyone interested in pursuing it must submit an investigational new drug (IND) application for approval. The FDA letter states that any "human cells used in therapy involving the transfer of genetic material by means other than the union of gamete nuclei" is subject to its strict regulations. A spokeswoman for the FDA says this is because these techniques are "types of gene therapy."

"They call it gene therapy because mitochondrial DNA is involved. It's the most ridiculous definition of gene therapy that I've ever heard," says Dr. James Grifo, who was the first to get an FDA letter. Victoria Girard, an attorney for the ASRM, agrees to some extent. She believes the FDA has a role to play, but says it remains unclear whether this is gene therapy, or that the resulting embryos should be considered investigational drugs. "You have to always remember that in our country, the right to reproductive freedom is one of those kinds of fundamental sacred rights, and every time you encroach on that, you need to be thinking very carefully about the policy implications and everything else related to it. I don't think the FDA should come in and do it just because they can do it, without thinking it through."

The major concern stems from the fact that some of the donor's mitochondrial DNA enters the same fertilized egg cell containing the mother and father's nuclear DNA, potentially producing a child with genes from *three* people. Further unease surfaced when scientists at St. Barnabas Medical Center in New Jersey reported that two of their cytoplasmic transfer pregnancies resulted in fetuses carrying a chromosomal abnormality. Though there is no direct evidence linking the abnormality to the mitochondrial DNA, anxiety over the procedure remains. Researchers in favor of the technique say it's not unusual to have chromosomal abnormalities in the infertile population; they see them all the time. As in this case, the pregnancies are usually either terminated or end in miscarriage. Others say it's too soon to know for sure.

Published reports indicate these young children are healthy and normal, and in the case of the St. Barnabas children, only two of the children reportedly have any mitochondrial DNA from the donor cytoplasm. The Fakih clinic in Lebanon produced seven children using cytoplasmic transfer before receiving the FDA letter. Sharon Saarinen had one of those babies. She feels extremely fortunate she went to Dr. Michael Fakih's clinic when she did, otherwise she is sure she would be childless. "I don't think it's a fluke that I got pregnant with this cytoplasm procedure. It's [the] only thing that worked for me."

Sharon had failed five attempts at traditional IVF because she always produced just a few nonviable eggs. On her first try with cytoplasmic transfer, her daughter Alana was conceived. She says her daughter is perfect in every way, and has passed every developmental milestone ahead of schedule. She even went back to the clinic a year later to try for a second child, but was told they could no longer offer the technique. She's angry and frustrated over the FDA's restrictions. "I think it's a shame that this option no longer exists, because it works. I have a healthy, happy, intelligent child thanks to this procedure. I feel so blessed to have her."

While Fakih has turned his sights toward self-cytoplasmic transfer, Grifo hopes to continue to pursue his nuclear transfer research. He intends to submit an IND application to the FDA, though he says it is extremely time consuming and prohibitively expensive. "We simply don't have the resources of the large drug companies. But they're calling me a drug maker—I make drugs called embryos, I put them in patients, so now I am regulated like a major drug company—a multibillion dollar corporation versus a little academic shoestring budget. But we're going to try." It remains to be seen whether the FDA will grant any clinics or institutions approval to continue the research.

The Future of the Biological Clock

It's already possible to freeze your eggs, and within the next decade, you will likely be assured of even higher success rates. But that's not all. One day it may also be possible to make eggs from any cell in your body, because you will be able to produce a cloned embryo to make the stem cells, which can then make your eggs. If further science reveals there are stem cells in your ovaries, a minor biopsy would enable you to make a potentially endless supply of *your own* viable eggs at any age.

However, there are other likely developments to help keep your clock ticking as long as you would like. Some forward thinkers see a day when women will take a simple pill to put their ovaries on hold or keep them working as long as they would like. This medication might simply turn off the clock for awhile, so you can start it up again when you decide rather than sit idly by as mother nature zaps you of your fertility leaving you with no way to do anything about it. This would also mean staving off menopause and possibly all the health risks that go along with it—osteoporosis, heart disease, depression. Of course, those who would prefer an earlier menopause once they have their children would also be able to stop the clock indefinitely.

At the very least, unscrambling the genetic code of menopause will provide a much clearer look at the biological clock, so women know how long they have before their fertility declines and menopause commences, giving them greater flexibility in planning families and careers, *without* biomedical intervention. This, combined with more precise ways to determine egg count, and possibly stem

184

cell count and viability, will permit even better reproductive life span calculations.

Those who argue that this is ridiculous—an affront on Mother Nature, likely haven't felt the pain, distress, and devastation of a biological clock that has quit precisely when your lifelong dream of children is supposed to be coming true. If these possibilities are unnatural, then so be it. One could make the argument that so is all of medicine. It is unnatural to perform a heart transplant, give chemotherapy, and provide morphine at the end of life. If improving the lives of countless women (and men) through future technology by allowing them more freedom to pursue one of the most innate biological functions, most intense human desires, and the only way to ensure survival of our species is unnatural, then I, along with many others, say, "Go for it!"

GOLDEN MOTHERING

8.

Then God said, "Yes, but your wife Sarah will bear you a son, and you will call him Isaac."

—Genesis 17:19

Nothing New

Having children later in life is as ancient as the Bible's Old Testament. In this passage, God was speaking to Abraham, who was 100 years old, and whose wife, Sarah, was a spry 90! Abraham had been able to have a child previously, though the married couple had so far not been able to have a child together. Interestingly, several years earlier, Sarah helped her husband have a child through an arrangement with her Egyptian maidservant. According to the book of Genesis 16:1–4, this first biblical form of egg donation/surrogacy, produced a baby boy called Ishmael.

It appears from this bible story that age played little role in God's decision to help this infertile couple finally have a child. The birth of Isaac was considered a miracle, as would a spontaneous birth to a 90-year-old woman today. However, with current medical techniques, an egg donor, and a very fit 90-year-old, amazingly enough, this story could be repeated. It would no doubt be called a miracle, but today, rather than celebrated, the mother would likely be scorned, perhaps even publicly ridiculed, for becoming a parent at such a golden age.

Older Parents on the Rise

It may be quite some time before nonagenarians become mothers on a routine basis, but today across the civilized world, more older women than ever are becoming mothers, many for the first time. In the United States and much of Western society, the only group of women with rising birth rates are those over age 35. Teenage births are continuously declining, births to young 20-somethings are dropping, babies born to those 25- to 34-years-old are largely unchanged, but births to those 35 or over have consistently climbed annually according to the National Vital Statistics Reports of the CDC. In fact, the birth rate (41 births for every 1,000 women) for women 35 to 39, and the birth rate (eight births for every 1,000 women) for those ages 40 to 44, are the highest in more than 30 years. The latest statistics also reveal the average age for a first birth is now over 25, the oldest ever recorded in the United States. In 1970 the average was just 21.4 years. For the record, Massachusetts has the highest average age for first-time moms at 28; this is also the state with the most comprehensive mandated insurance coverage for infertility.

Similar findings have been reported in other Western societies. In Great Britain there are now more first-time mothers over age 30 than under 25, and the number of mothers over 40 also continues to rise. A review of older motherhood written by a group in Australia reported that the median age for childbearing is rising and the birth rate for women older than 35 is growing faster than for any other age group.

The trends are clear, more women are choosing to become mothers later in life, and more children are now born to older parents than ever before. These statistics also likely reflect many more planned pregnancies than later-in-life surprises; they may also mirror the most motivated hopeful mothers and fathers who have struggled with a less than adequate female biological clock to achieve a very wanted child. It is therefore reasonable to conclude that *more* babies would likely be born to older parents were it not for the difficulties of fertility treatment as well as the often insurmountable financial roadblocks. It's no secret, and by now you are likely aware, that unprecedented numbers of reproductively older women are flocking to reproductive medicine clinics for help having children.

Serious Problem or Quaint Social Phenomenon?

Many countries have raised substantial concerns regarding this later-in-life parenthood trend. Why? The more older moms, the fewer children added to the population. Researchers in Denmark have published data showing the average number of babies born to a woman over her lifetime is now less than two in many European countries including the United Kingdom, Denmark, Finland, Sweden, Germany, Italy, Spain, as well as in Japan. They claim that at this rate, these countries will be unable to sustain current population levels. This could bode trouble for future generations: a substantially lowered tax base, fewer services, fewer jobs, and less ability to support their elderly citizens and keep the wheels of society turning.

Researchers at the Vienna Institute of Demography calculate that if the current trend continues, there will be 88 million fewer people in Europe at the turn of the next century. A situation that they write in *Science* magazine, "…may hinder productivity gains, and could affect global competitiveness and economic growth." This group suggests immediate changes to help reverse the population decline, such as social and employment policies to encourage women to have children sooner, though they admit, such policies have had little effect in the past. Many experts believe something has to be done.

In the United States the situation is not nearly as dire, thanks to our ethnic diversity. Though many women are opting for later motherhood, and hence fewer children, they are generally white Americans. The U.S. Census Bureau shows population growth among Caucasians is slowing, whereas it is growing rapidly among minorities, especially amid Hispanics and Asians. Census Bureau projections show the population will nearly double over the next 50 years, due mostly to the birth and immigration rates of minorities. This will certainly change the face of America, because by 2050, minority groups are expected to become close to 50 percent of the population. Adjustments will undoubtedly be made to U.S. society; however, it doesn't appear that we are headed for major threats to infrastructure akin to Europe due to deficient numbers.

Behind the Trend

Social Changes

The most obvious reason women are delaying childbearing is because they are busy working, building careers, and becoming productive members of society. It just so happened that the explosion in educational and career opportunities for women coincided with the advent of the birth control pill. The ability to control reproduction and pursue a profession has resulted in unprecedented numbers of women seeking to become mothers in their mid- to late 30s and 40s. Included in this group are many women who for one reason or another meet their mates later in life as well. In my inner circle of friends and family, I can rattle off several women who have finally met their soul mates at 40 or older. One of my best friends, a corporate executive, just married for the first time at age 45. My cousin, after years of dating frogs, finally met her prince at age 47. I, on the other hand, stumbled onto my true love just in time to use my last good egg—at age 39. In addition, many people want to have a child during their second marriage. The bottom line is pursuing careers, striving for financial security, meeting mates later, and second marriages are driving this golden age baby boom.

Living Longer, Living Better

How long do you expect to live? Currently in the United States the life expectancy for a woman is 79.8 years. Given how much healthier middle-aged women are today, and knowing they, on average, could make it to nearly 80, it's easy to see why many want children in their late 30s, 40s, some even in their 50s. In fact, researchers are now finding that more women than ever might even have the natural ability to produce children later in life. Thomas Perls, M.D., of Boston University School of Public Health, has studied the oldest of the old, and has found that those reaching 100 years of age are the fastest growing segment of the population, the second fastest are those reaching 85 or older. As you may expect, there are far more female centenarians than male, at 90 percent versus 10 percent, respectively.

Most intriguing is that Perls has also discovered that women who live the longest also tend to have babies the latest—naturally. When he reviewed the centenarian subjects in the suburban Boston area, he found a substantial number of women who had children in their 40s, and one even in her early 50s. Further review of the data showed that more than 19 percent of the centenarians had children in their 40s compared to just 5.5 percent of the women used as controls, who lived to just 73 years old. Perls and his team concluded that having a child after age 40 may not confer longevity, but it may indicate a slower reproductive clock and the likelihood that a woman will live a very long life. They calculated that an over-40 mother is four times more likely to survive to 100 than age 73.

Donor Eggs

Women who are destined for centenarian status may not need help if they decide to have a midlife baby, but many others who are less fortunate must turn to medicine and often a younger woman for assistance. Perhaps the greatest advance in the treatment for older hopeful mothers is the ability to use donated eggs to create a child. Until doctors attempted this technique, it was unclear whether the problem with a sluggish biological clock would be found within the ovaries, uterus, hormonal communications system, or any combination thereof. It became almost immediately apparent, however, that the eggs and therefore the ovaries were the culprit in reproductively older women. Barring any uterine problems, if you replace old eggs with young ones, the chances of successful pregnancy skyrockets.

Who uses donor eggs? Many younger women use donor eggs; these are usually women headed for an earlier menopause who lose their fertility in their 30s, or those who for one reason or another produce poor-quality eggs. However, the number of donor cycles performed jumps exponentially starting at age 39, with just about all using donor eggs at 45 or older. It's easy to see why. The CDC's data shows the live birth rate for women at this age is next to zero when using their own eggs, but remains on par with much younger women when donor eggs are used; this is true even for women who are already meno-pausal. So, it stands to reason that if a couple's goal is to have a child, the chances are far greater with donor eggs than with the woman's own *older* eggs.

Pushing the Limits

Exactly how old is too old to become a mother? Biologically, we really don't know the extreme limit. At the moment, the oldest woman to gestate and give birth to a baby is a 65-year-old retired school-teacher from India. According to published reports, the baby boy weighed in at 6 pounds 8 ounces, was delivered by C-section, and was conceived through eggs donated by the mother's 26-year-old niece. Prior to this birth, two women tied for the "oldest" mother status: one came from Italy, the other, southern California, both were 63 years old and also used younger donor eggs.

These cases prove without a doubt that donor eggs can allow nearly any woman in good health to spend her retirement years caring for a newborn and raising a child. It is important to note, however, that the oldest woman on record to have conceived with her own egg and car-ried a baby to term was 57 years old, according to the *Guinness Book of World Records*. The Portland, Oregon, woman gave birth to a daugh-ter in 1956, long before medicine figured out a way to reset the clock by using donor eggs. This record has stood for nearly half a century, so although it is *possible* for a 57-year-old to have a baby, so far a natural conception and birth at 57 has been documented in only *one* woman.

A recent study, however, has shown that women's bodies are very resilient when it comes to gestating a fetus, even following menopause. Basically, if you have the incubator—that is, a uterus—all it may need is a hormonal tune-up to get back into working order. Richard Paulson, M.D., chief of the division of Reproductive Endocrinology and Infer-tility at the University of Southern California School of Medicine, led the study that showed that women in their 50s can successfully have babies through egg donation. "I'm, of course, very comfortable with it now, but when we were first talking about treating women over 50, I thought 'geez!'" Paulson says his initial reluctance stemmed from reproductive norms that were about to be turned upside down. "When

192

I was a resident at the fertility clinic at the county hospital, they didn't take women over 40, that was too old, period."

Paulson treated the 63-year-old woman who remains the oldest U.S. woman to become a mother. Once she became pregnant, she revealed her true age. It turned out she had claimed to be 53, and her medical records reflected that untruth. Otherwise she would have been turned away from Paulson's clinic. Ironically, her pregnancy has helped establish more comprehensive data on pregnancy outcomes in older women in the scientific literature. Because Paulson and his team have treated so many over-50 women using donated eggs, they have led the way in this kind of research.

The most definitive findings to date show that in pregnant women age 50 or older, there is a higher rate of hypertension, preeclampsia, and gestational diabetes compared to younger women. For instance, pregnancy-induced hypertension was 10 times more likely in women over 50 than much younger women, and three times more likely than in women over 40. The team also showed an even higher risk of both hypertension and gestational diabetes in women over 55 compared to those aged 50 to 54. Paulson says the study has provided a kind of age guidepost for clinics. "It looks like at 55 we may have inadvertently hit the physiological limit—at least at the present time and with present obstetrical techniques and our understanding of disease."

Still, with careful obstetrical care, at least one woman has been able to add 10 years to Paulson's documented physiologically *safe* boundary. There's every reason to believe someone, somewhere will push that limit further.

Older Moms Tell Their Stories

This life would not exist without me. That means something to me at some fundamental level. I can look at my sweet daughter and say, "I created this beautiful thing."

—Lauren, 45, used donor eggs

Considering we'll be 68 and 73, when our child goes to college— we're not at the ends of our working lives per se, but we'll probably have to continue working to come up with college tuition.

—Rhonda, 50, used donor eggs

What Every Woman Needs to Know About...Her Biological Clock

*Most of my relatives lived into their 80s and 90s, even with poor
lifestyle habits and medical problems, so the way I see it,
I still have half my life before me.
Why shouldn't I spend it raising a family if I want to?*

—The author, 43, talking to her doctor

We are the ageless generation. Have you seen Cher lately? Tell me that woman is pushing 60! I caught Christy Brinkley on a morning talk show recently, and she admits she's almost 50, though she hardly looks 32. Men may not battle the wrinkles, but they're faring just as well—Mick Jagger belts out a Stones classic with as much energy as he did 30 years ago; even Tony Bennett is still performing, and bringing down the house at nearly 80! Is it any wonder that women and men alike feel as though they cannot only look young, but also do what young people do—for instance, have children?

Take our youth-driven society and mix a little false information about advances in reproductive medicine, or equally ruinous, leave out the dose of biological clock reality, and you come up with a brew that compels people to believe they have a lot more time to have children. Once they walk into a reproductive medicine clinic and are offered an alternative to their own reproductive capacity—the ability to create a child through the use of younger donor eggs—they may initially reject the idea, but eventually begin to acquire a taste for it, and lo and behold their original assumptions begin to hold true. They *can* have a child, at a time in their lives when in all of previous human history they would have remained childless.

Such was the case for Rhonda and Lauren. Both had their first child at what is considered to be *advanced maternal age*. They both accomplished this goal through the use of donor eggs, following many gut-wrenching struggles with trying to use their own eggs, and in Rhonda's case, even having several previous donor egg cycles and adoptions fail. Their stories complement each other well. Lauren is in her 40s, and Rhonda is in her 50s. Lauren got pregnant with her first attempt at donor; Rhonda struggled for many more years. Lauren is now pregnant with her second donor child; Rhonda tried to have a second, but failed, and now has no further options due to age and financial constraints.

Both women arrived at their golden motherhood via similar circumstances. They met their mates later in life, and thought they had

194

more time to have their own genetic children. Rhonda married at age 44 and figured she had at least another five years, because she knew her female relatives went through menopause at around age 50. She based her family planning on lack of information about the biological clock. Having been pregnant and miscarried a couple of times also boosted her confidence; a typical "glass is half full" response, when often, miscarriages later in life signal that the glass is likely half empty.

Following a very poor response to stimulation and IVF, she decided to try using an egg donor. This initial attempt failed. She and her husband then tried to adopt. Their first try failed. On their second effort, the birth mother changed her mind. And on the third, after traveling halfway across the country to attend the birth, care for the newborn in the hospital, and fall in love with him, the birth mother left the hospital with the baby. Devastated, Rhonda returned home empty-handed. At that point she decided to find another egg donor, and went to a different clinic because she was now past the age limit for her previous clinic. That attempt failed as well, and soon after, the clinic closed. Finally, she went to a New Jersey clinic that would accommodate her, and became pregnant with her daughter on her first try. She was two months shy of her 50th birthday when Sophia was born.

Now she can't even imagine life without her. "She's changed it completely. My personality has changed, I am a much more nurturing person than I ever used to be." With all she's gone through, Rhonda feels as though she should have 10 kids rather than just one, but even one completely fills a void. "I have had some moments of pure joy with my daughter in a way that I have never experienced before."

It took Lauren nearly as long to have her first child, although she started sooner. She married at age 36, and tried to get pregnant for a long time on her own and then with traditional IVF before turning to a donor at age 42. She remembers always being told her chances were slim due to her high FSH even in her late 30s. She also recalls being revolted at the idea of using someone else's eggs to have a child. However, after much soul-searching, and grieving over the loss of the child she thought she would have, she realized that she wanted a *child* more than she wanted a child in her own image. She advertised and found an egg donor on her own, and at the age of 43, her daughter Alissa was born; she became pregnant recently through a frozen embryo cycle, and will be 45 when her second child—Alissa's genetic sibling—is born.

For Lauren, finally having a family is a dream come true, "This is the best thing I ever did. I feel like a have a full life now. I didn't for a long time, and I didn't even know it."

Society's Dichotomous Comfort Level

Although more women are having children later, society is a long way from accepting motherhood at midlife and beyond. When I was pregnant with my son, I remember a conversation with a colleague on the way to our assignment, where age and parenthood came up. He said something to the effect of, "I don't know why someone would want to have a child at 40; at that point they should just give it up." He had no idea I was 40! Of course when I told him, he was shocked. After I told him why I still wanted a family, I think he understood. Five years later, I bumped into him again while eight months pregnant with my second; he simply congratulated me.

This kind of thinking is pervasive within the general population, especially among those who have zero experience with either a loved one or friend who, for whatever reason, came to want and/or have children later in life. If people recoil at women having children at 40, what about 45, 50, or now even over 60? Bioethicist Paul Wolpe says women are caught in a kind of reproduction catch-22, "It's a double-edged sword. Women are being told to have children later, and now they are having them later, and it's not such a great thing."

But men have been fathering children at those ages for eons. My dad was one of them. He was 55 when I was born, and 60 when my younger *twin* sisters were born—and he was a hero. Had my mother given birth to twins at 60, she likely would have been ridiculed as selfish, caring more for her own desires than her children's future. As it turns out, so far she's made it to 78, he died at 72. So who would have been better off having kids at 60? Obviously, there are many factors to consider, but the fact is, I was 16 and my sisters were only 12 when we lost our dad; we would have had our mom around for many more years had she been the one to have us so much later in life.

The media also applauds older fathers, sometimes referred to as "dinosaur dads." Woody Allen, Warren Beatty, and Larry King became fathers in their 60s; Charlie Chaplin, Tony Randall, and Anthony Quinn had children in their 70s; Anthony Quinn became a father again at 81, and according to reports, Julio Iglesias's father is expecting a son at 87. That means Julio will have a brother 60 years his junior; and this newest addition will become an uncle to 10 nieces and nephews, including heartthrob Enrique. These dads are celebrated, praised, even admired by society for their virility. Their obituaries don't even point out the fact that they have left very young children behind. Wolpe says it's a double standard, based on a widely held assumption. "People emotionally expect women to take care of the children. So when mothers are not going to be around, people think it's bad. They don't expect fathers to be the primary caretaker."

Pros and Cons of Golden Motherhood

Obviously, society and its children would suffer if 60-, 70-, and 80-year-old women began having children with similarly aged fathers. I understand firsthand the difficulty older parenthood brings. My dad missed our high school graduations, our college graduations, our weddings, and children. Is this any different for older mothers? In fact, older mothers with younger fathers may be more advantageous for children, because statistically, women live longer than men. The societal assumption that women should be younger to be around longer may make sense on some visceral level, however, let's not forget that traditionally, men have always been the providers. When my dad died, his business folded, and my mother had no way to replace the income we had depended on. My mom had four young children to support, and little to no financial resources to do so. The supposition that older fathers who leave young children have little impact is a false one.

Rhonda is quick to point out the drawbacks to being older for both she and her husband. "We need to be saving for retirement, and we need to be saving for college, and we're having a hard time doing either of those." She says this sobering fact is also preventing them from having a second, and giving their daughter a sibling. At the same time, she's finding less in common with her friends who are now empty-nesters. Finally, Rhonda wonders about her daughter's relationship with older relatives. "I never thought about picturing my child at her wedding, and wondering who was going to be around to invite."

Lauren has similar concerns about the future. "The time that we have with her is so precious; we live our lives from that perspective, and that's probably a good thing for her." However, she sees many more advantages to having a family later rather than sooner. First, she and her husband are financially secure because they are both well established in their careers. "I can be calm about this, and if I were younger, when I was still trying to prove something, I couldn't be." Also, she believes maturity is a blessing. "I think my daughter is getting more out of her upbringing because of where I am in life, and I think I am too. I might have had more physical stamina in my 20s, but I was not at all emotionally equipped to be a mother in those days, no question about it." As for impressions of those who oppose older motherhood, "one of the other benefits of being a little bit older is that you just don't care what people think anymore."

Setting Limits

The use of donor eggs has shattered any traditional idea of the perfect age for mothering. Now the sky is the limit. But just because it's possible to become a mother at any age, should we? For men, the same questions holds, only there are no questionnaires to fill out, medical exams to pass, or thresholds to cross before they can be granted permission to undergo child-producing treatments. As long as they have viable sperm and a willing fertile mate, a man can become a father at any age. It's not that easy for older women.

About half the reproductive medicine clinics I researched set an age limit for providing donor egg services. Some are as low as 45, the highest is 55. Those that do not have age cutoffs take patients on a case-by-case basis. So it's not out of the question that a very fit 57- or 58-year-old could be treated, although, with few exceptions, the doctors I spoke with said they would be reluctant to treat anyone past the age of 60. Pat McShane, M.D., director of the Reproductive Science Center just outside of Boston refuses most women past the age of 45, and makes few exceptions. "People don't think beyond the first five years of life and they don't realize what level of energy and involvement is going to be required of them when the child is 14, 16, and 20. That is one of the things I do have a lot of concern about."

On the other hand, Richard Paulson, M.D., relies on the scientific data he's collected on the obstetrical risks older women face, and sets his California clinic's age limit at 55. He has made exceptions, though he denied a woman who had twins at 54, and wanted to try again at 57. "I said, you've got two, I'm sorry, we're not going to do it." But he does leave the option open, and says, "If somebody should walk through that door at 57, and they are the editor of longevity magazine, and they run marathons, and they look 40—maybe it will be all right."

Who Should Decide?

It's clear that it's usually not up to the woman or her husband whether they can become parents past a certain age. This decision generally rests with the clinic director and/or her doctor. These are the reproductive gatekeepers; and they say no all the time. Is this right?

Professor of health law, bioethics, and human rights at Boston University School of Public Health, George Annas, J.D., MPH, says, "No." He believes doctors shouldn't be setting age limits. "Obviously, you have to go through a lot to get these kids, so as long as you really want to be a parent, not just have a kid, but really want to raise a child, it's hard to make any ethical argument against it." Annas says the standpoint that it's too risky to gestate the child and give birth doesn't hold up well, either. "The answer to that is to hire somebody to do it. There are some ethical problems there, but the main problem is not age, whenever you look at these things, it's not going to be age."

Colleague Michael Grodin, M.D., professor and director of the Law, Medicine, and Ethics Program at BU, tends to agree, especially given how much these children are wanted. "It is much more detrimental to have a parent that doesn't want the kid, doesn't love the kid, than it is to have a parent who wants, loves, cares for the child, and then drops dead."

Both ethicists agree that it is unethical to set limits based solely on age. Annas argues, "Any age cutoff is arbitrary, and so you have to have some data to back it up, some reason—not just that you don't like it, that it's a personal preference. Society sure hasn't come up with a rule, so doctors are making one up." Grodin suggests, "At minimum, clinics have to be open and clear and explicit about what the rules are and how they came up with them, and they have to be verifiable."

Some doctors, on the other hand, feel a tremendous amount of responsibility when making such life versus *no* life decisions. "We, as physicians, have to take care of all the individuals involved. We have to take care of the donor, we have to take care of the recipient, and we have to take care of the baby, and they're all equal participants, and they all have equal rights," says Zev Rosenwaks, M.D. He restricts donor egg services to women of reproductive age based on safety to the mother and child. He says women over age 50 are not eligible for the program, and adds, "Recognizing that one can't predict in life, but certainly, the fear and maybe terror of having very old parents—one can see easily that presents a problem for a child, and the problem is not just theoretical, for the child it can be very real."

Linda Applegarth, Ed.D., director of Psychological Services at Rosenwaks's clinic, worries about the implications for children of much older parents. "Obviously, I have no data, but what if you leave your child an orphan? You had a child at 55, and at 70 your dead—all of a sudden you have a 15-year-old who is missing one or both parents, or is having to deal with aging parents or parents who are ill, at a very young age."

David Keefe, M.D., director of clinics in Boston and Providence, Rhode Island, refuses to set any age limit. "We do it case by case. We make sure they are healthy whatever age they are, and they've thought it through." Keefe points to his mother who had her last child at 47, and remained healthy and sharp until she died suddenly at 91. "That's how it is for many people, conversely some people get Alzheimer's at 40—it's such a presumptuous thing to set age limits. I know many women who are now 50, who have another 30 to 35 years of very good living."

He also relies on his psychiatry background to fortify his position. "Obviously, if somebody was a serial killer, had convictions for child abuse, a pedophile, yes, that's a problem. There are certain circumstances where somebody's not suitable. But short of that?" He is also opposed to age limits based on health risks to the mother because the patient is always informed about them, they can be monitored and treated with good obstetrical care, and such policies are not in place for younger women who can have the same complications.

Keefe insists reproductive freedom holds whether you are doing technology or not. "People sort of assume that we are creating life and we're playing God and so therefore we have to be like God and make the rules, and that's not at all the case; we're just facilitating it, and the rules that apply are still pretty much the same rules that apply in a natural conception, and you don't go around making rules about that."

As a daughter of an older father, I can understand the concerns of those opposed to older parenthood, but, make no mistake, I'm still glad I'm here. As for grandparents, I never knew my father's parents; my mother's parents died when I was in college, both in their 80s; my son and new daughter will never know my father; my son's namesake grandfather is 88, and both grandmothers are 78. All are in fairly good health and should be around for some time.

Who Should Pay?

If our fundamental rights are life, liberty, and the *pursuit of happiness*, shouldn't having children be covered? Isn't that why people want children—to bless them with the kind of joy unique to this human endeavor? There is no other pleasure in life (and this comes from someone who had a very exciting, professionally rewarding, fun-filled, adventurous, happy 20 years of single life) that compares with having a child. None. Period.

What does this have to do with money? Plainly, the vast majority of those who discover they are infertile in the United States must pay for all of their medical expenses out of pocket. And it doesn't matter how old you are. When I first sought a reproductive medicine clinic and contacted my insurance company, they told me some diagnostic tests would be covered, but not treatment. I nearly fell over. I live in Massachusetts, which has the most comprehensive infertility coverage in the country, and where my colleagues had assured me that their infertility treatment was completely covered. Still, my insurer said they would cover me to find out what's wrong, but wouldn't pay to fix it. Hmmmm. Seems to me that's like having an X-ray, and the doctor telling you, "You've got a broken leg, but sorry, no cast, just let it flop around—oh, and be aware you will walk with a limp for the rest of your life." This makes no sense, especially because I knew something was wrong—I had just had a baby one year prior. Make no mistake, not being able to treat infertility is a lot worse than a limp, you might as well cut off the entire leg!

The reason I wasn't covered for treatment—even in Massachusetts— has to do with a federal law that exempts private insurers from covering

201

state-mandated treatments. At the time, although I was working full time (and then some) at the TV station, I received my health insurance through my union, the American Federation of Television and Radio Artists (AFTRA). So although I was working for the same company, others who received coverage through the local station were covered, but because AFTRA is a private group insurer, I was not! Of course, this news came right when I had zero time to waste, and needed treatment immediately. Most of America experiences this sudden financial roadblock when it comes to infertility; however, in my situation, I was surrounded by a sea of people who had options, including multiple IVF cycles, whereas I felt the financial pressure equivalent of an armada of big rigs falling on my head!

Obviously this situation has to be changed. As of 2003, multiple federal bills have been proposed to force insurance companies to provide coverage for reproductive medicine, specifically ART. One would undo the damage done by the federal law that allowed AFTRA to deny me coverage, even though I work and live in a state that mandates full infertility coverage. This law would remove exemption status for private insurers operating in such states. It is important to note that currently, only 15 states provide either coverage or at least an offer to cover infertility. That's why the Family Building Act of 2003 is so important. It requires coverage for the treatment of infertility, or the inability to carry a pregnancy to a live birth; it mandates *all* insurers covering obstetrical services include infertility treatment.

Other bills currently in process would require Medicare to pay for infertility treatments for those who are eligible for benefits, as well as all health plans available to federal employees, and the military and their families. Currently, a soldier can risk his life in the War on Terror, but faces an uphill battle accessing and paying for aggressive infertility treatments if he and his wife need help having a family. Contraceptives, however, are covered. Sometimes what is covered and what's not make absolutely no sense. So another federal bill has been introduced to force all insurers who provide coverage for Viagra and other impotence drugs to also cover infertility treatments. The Equity in Fertility Coverage Act of 2003, essentially says that if you're paying to fix men's erections, then you must pay for women to have babies.

At the most fundamental of levels, it only makes sense that infertility treatment be covered by health insurance plans. This disease affects one out of every 10 couples—that's 6 million people in the

United States. In most circumstances, only those who can afford 10s of thousands of dollars out of pocket will be able to access the proven treatment that offers the best chance for a success. Insurers argue that such federal laws, if passed, would force healthcare costs to sky-rocket. However, a Massachusetts study found that the cost of cover-age was one of the lowest among its mandated benefits at just $2.49 per member per year. Hardly worth arguing over, given the potential benefits to all citizens as well as society in general.

Speaking of benefits, let's not forget that these are extremely wanted children, who are loved and provided for both emotionally and finan-cially. The costs surely can't outweigh the potential advantages to bringing these children into the world. Also, many believe covering infertility procedures will actually reduce expenditures for costly ob-stetrical care, births, and potential lifelong health coverage for mul-tiple gestations and births, because patients and doctors will be less likely to dole out Clomid unmonitored, or transfer multiple embryos for IVF.

Because people must pay out of pocket, many feel compelled to use as many embryos as the doctors will allow. This gives couples the highest chance to succeed, with less risk of future costs *to them* for further cycles. Once a pregnancy takes hold, insurance must cover it. The high incidence of multiple gestations and births increases the amount any insurance company has to pay. Even a twin pregnancy can mean hundreds of thousands of dollars for monitoring and hospi-tal stays if there are complications. A triplet birth can cost upwards of $340,000. The higher rate of preterm births requiring neonatal inten-sive care, and perhaps additional care for physical or cognitive devel-opmental delays also increases the expense.

Finally, the emotional toll exacted by the inability to have a child is immeasurable. Most insurers will cover the cost of mental health services, including anxiety and depression, which accompanies in-fertility. The hope ART can provide alleviates some of this distress, and if successful, can totally eliminate the need for any further men-tal health support. Coverage for ART would alleviate a tremendous amount of suffering among the most productive members of soci-ety, with the added bonus of bringing more productive and future taxpayers into the world.

What About Age?

It's pretty easy to make the case for a federal insurance mandate to cover infertility. However, there remains the question of age, and whether treatment for age-related infertility, or (the term I hate) *impaired ovarian reserve*, should be included in such coverage. After all, isn't it just a part of growing older that our biological clocks wind down? Should private and group insurance plans, Medicare, or the government pay for treatment to overcome a natural biological process? It is a sticky question, especially given that medicine *can* tune up, even replace parts, and turn over the engine of an obsolete biological clock.

Simple answer is yes; otherwise, insurers run the risk of sliding down that slippery slope called age discrimination. It would be difficult to deny a 40-year-old woman ART, but cover a 35-year-old. However, even in states where infertility is covered, that is already beginning to happen. In Massachusetts, women are not only being denied based on age (45 appears to be a major cutoff), but they are being turned down based on ovarian reserve tests. Often, if there is a delay, even for a medical reason, insurance companies are requiring another FSH or Clomid Challenge Test before granting coverage extensions. Everyone knows the news can only get worse with time. Insurers are now using elevated FSH results to deny coverage, even when there is still a chance for a pregnancy.

In my case, I finally accessed health coverage that included infertility treatment, and applied for IVF. I was refused based on an elevated Clomid Challenge Test they forced me to take. So, even though I finally found a way to access health coverage by paying the premiums out of pocket, I was never able to do IVF with my own eggs. I was devastated. My doctor suggested we request a donor cycle. Figuring I had nothing to lose, we did, and it was granted. However, the insurer gave me a seven-month deadline, which ended exactly one day before my 44th birthday. After I had four donors fall through and realized I would not make that deadline, my insurer requested another Clomid Challenge Test! I refused to do it, and asked my doctor to simply request another two months, because I had finally found a great donor and was set to begin the procedure. The insurance company relented, and I got pregnant. Thank goodness.

Why put people through this? The treatment exists, it works, and still couples must go through hell to bring a child into the world. If I had coverage to begin with, I may have been successful sooner, wouldn't have required two years of counseling that the insurance company paid for, and would have been off the books much quicker. I am grateful that at least we had some options and enough fighting spirit to accomplish our goal. Most others are not as fortunate. Without options, there is nothing to fight for.

Bioethicist Paul Wolpe believes strongly that infertility should be covered, and agrees there should be some limitations based on age, but he has a fairly straightforward resolution. "You solve the problem the same way you do in life insurance. You want to give cheaper life insurance to people who are 20 than people who are 60. It isn't that you deny the 45-year-old infertility insurance, you just make them pay a premium for it—so you have an age-rated insurance policy. I don't think it's immoral to help a 45-year-old to have a child, I don't think it's necessarily immoral to help a 55-year-old have a child, just like if a 55-year-old man came in with a low motility [sperm] problem, we would help that person."

In a perfect world, people who want to have a child would be able to access the care and treatment that would help them do so regardless of age. Let's not forget that every other age-related ailment is covered by insurance, even those brought on by the patients themselves. Insurers cover major heart surgery that can be directly linked to poor diet and lifestyle; emphysema brought on by decades of smoking; they also replace countless joints that have deteriorated due to extended use. Some argue that covering fertility treatment in older women is akin to paying for plastic surgery. Need I go there? A baby vs. a face-lift, hmmmm, are these people nuts? Just more confirmation that we will never live in a perfect world.

Wolpe's recommendation represents a possible compromise. At the very least it would give more people the opportunity to try to have a child, not just those in the tip-top income brackets. I would not be looking forward to the birth of my second child, exactly one week from today, if I had no infertility insurance coverage. We nevertheless spent a substantial amount out of pocket to accomplish our goal because we had to pay an agency, lawyers, compensate a donor, and pay high premiums each month. But if the treatment hadn't been covered, we simply could not have afforded it. Ultimately, my health plan still tried to slam the door on my coverage, but I hung on, and kept it open just enough to slip through the crack. A testament that *any* option can make all the difference in the world.

Final Word

Understanding your biological clock brings you one step closer to beating it. All of the information contained in the previous pages is meant to help you devise a plan so that you can have all that life has to offer, including children. It is likely you have realized that the earlier you start this plan, the easier it will be to implement it. Anyone who has faced a compromised biological clock, and still wants children, will tell you there is no easy, or inexpensive, way to do so. My wish and the main purpose of this book is to help many young women avoid this life-altering experience, by planning sooner and having children even just a little bit younger.

However, I know that is unrealistic. The relentless clock will continue to tick, while countless numbers of you, due to life circumstances, will be unable to start a family in time. Despite this information, you may eventually find yourself at the doorstep of a reproductive medicine clinic. Therefore, the previous pages are also filled with the most comprehensive information available in one source for you. I have strived to present everything, positive and less so, that I experienced and learned through my mission toward completing my family. It is not meant to frighten, only to inform. I truly hope it helps you better navigate through the sometimes rough waters you may encounter on your way to your future child's sparkling eyes and open arms.

RESOURCES

General Fertility Information

American Society for Reproductive Medicine
J. Benjamin Younger Office of Public Affairs
409 12th Street SW, Suite 203
Washington, DC 20024-2188
Tel: (202) 863-2494
Fax: (202) 484-4039
Search their Website for comprehensive fertility information: *www.asrm.org.*

Centers for Disease Control (CDC)
Assisted Reproductive Technology Reports: *www.cdc.gov/reproductivehealth/art.htm.*
Assisted Reproductive Technology Success Rates: Search the map to locate a clinic near you and compare success rates. *www.cdc.gov/reproductivehealth/ART01/index.htm.*

RESOLVE: The National Infertility Association
Search this Website for information and locate the chapter near you: *www.resolve.org.*

RESOLVE of the Baystate (Massachusetts)
9 Spring Street
PO Box 541553
Waltham, MA 02454-1553
Tel: (781) 647-1614
Fax: (781) 899-7207
Website: *www.resolveofthebaystate.org*
E-mail: admin@resolveofthebaystate.org

INCIID (The InterNational Council on Infertility Information Dissemination, Inc.)
PO Box 6836
Arlington, Virginia 22206
Tel: (703) 379-9178
Website: *www.inciid.org*
E-mail: information@inciid.org

American Infertility Association
Website: *www.americaninfertility.org*
Tel: (888) 917-3777

Egg-Freezing Information

Extend Fertility, Inc.
For information on egg freezing:
Tel: (800) 841-7197
Website: *www.extendfertility.com*
E-mail: info@extendfertility.com

Fertile Hope
For information on cancer treatments and fertility, and egg freezing:
PO Box 624
New York, NY 10014
Tel: (888) 994-HOPE
Website: *www.fertilehope.org*

Save My Eggs, Inc.
Website: *www.savemyeggs.com*

Community Health Network
Website: *www.ecommunity.com/assisted_fertility*

Help With High FSH

High FSH Message Board
Online support for those with high FSH: *www.network54.com/Forum/ 209394.*

Toxins Information

Environmental Working Group (EWG)
Washington Office
1436 U Street NW, Suite 100
Washington, DC 20009
Tel: (202) 667-6982
California Office
1904 Franklin #703
Oakland, CA 94612
Tel: (510) 444-0973
Search this site for toxic substances research: *www.ewg.org/reports/ bodyburden.*
Search this site for arsenic testing information: *www.ewg.org/reports/ poisonwoodrivals/orderform.php.*

U.S. Geological Survey
National Analysis of Trace Elements—Arsenic in Ground Water of the U.S.
See these Websites for maps and information on groundwater arsenic:
http://webserver.cr.usgs.gov/trace/pubs/geo_v46n11/fig3.html and
http://co.water.usgs.gov/trace.

U.S. Department of Labor Occupational Safety and Health Administration
200 Constitution Avenue, NW
Washington, DC 20210
Search these Websites for general toxins information:
www.osha.gov/dts/chemicalsampling/toc/toc_chemsamp.html
www.osha.gov/SLTC/hazaroustoxicsubstances/index.html
Search these Websites for information on fertility and pregnancy:
www.osha.gov/SLTC/reproductivehazards
www.cdc.gov/niosh/nrpreg.html

Other Selected Websites for Fertility Information

Protect Your Fertility Campaign: *www.protectyourfertility.org*

Association of Reproductive Health Professionals: *www.arhp.org*

American Pregnancy Association: *www.americanpregnancy.org*

Advanced Fertility Center of Chicago: *www.advancedfertility.com*

Boston IVF: *www.bostonivf.com*

The Center for Reproductive Medicine and Infertility: *www.ivf.org*

Huntington Reproductive Center: *www.havingbabies.com*

Jones Institute for Reproductive Medicine: *www.jonesinstitute.org*

Massachusetts General Hospital
The Vincent Center for Reproductive Biology:
www.massgeneral.org/depts/vcrb/vcrb_home.htm

Reproductive Science Center: *www.rscboston.com*

Women & Infants Hospital of Rhode Island
Division of Reproductive Medicine and Infertility:
www.womenandinfants.com

Select Bibliography

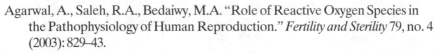

Agarwal, A., Saleh, R.A., Bedaiwy, M.A. "Role of Reactive Oxygen Species in the Pathophysiology of Human Reproduction." *Fertility and Sterility* 79, no. 4 (2003): 829–43.

American Infertility Association (AIA). "Fertility Survey Finds Astonishing Results: Only One of 12,382 Women Answered Correctly," press release, October 24, 2001, http://www.americaninfertility.org/media/ aia_survey_results.html.

American Society For Reproductive Medicine. *Age and Fertility, A Guide for Patients, 2003.*

ASRM Protect Your Fertility Campaign, booklet, *www.ProtectYourFertility.org.*

Barritt, J.A., C.A. Brenner, H.E. Malter, J. Cohen "Mitochondria in Human Offspring Derived From Ooplasmic Transplantation." *Human Reproduction* 16, no. 3 (2001): 513–6.

Battaglia, D.E., P. Goodwin, N.A. Klein, M.R. Soules. "Influence of Maternal Age on Meiotic Spindle Assembly in Oocytes From Naturally Cycling Women." *Human Reproduction* 11, no. 10 (1996): 2217–22.

Berga, S.L., T.L. Daniels, D.E. Giles. "Women With Functional Hypothalamic Amenorrhea but Not Other Forms of Anovulation Display Amplified Cortisol Concentrations." *Fertility and Sterility* 67, no. 6 (1997): 1024–30.

Berga, S.L., M.D. M arcus, T.L. Loucks, S. Hlastala, R. Ringham, M.A. Krohn. "Recovery of Ovarian Activity in Women With Functional Hypothalamic

Amenorrhea Who Were Treated With Cognitive Behavior Therapy." *Fertility and Sterility* 80, no. 4 (2003): 976–81.

Boldt, J., D. Cline, D. McLaughlin. "Human oocyte cryopreservation as an adjunct to IVF-embryo transfer cycles." *Human Reproduction* 18, no. 6 (2003): 1250–5.

Bolumar, F., J. Olsen, M. Rebagliato, L. Bisanti. "Caffeine Intake and Delayed Conception: A European Multicenter Study on Infertility and Subfecundity." European Study Group on Infertility Subfecundity. *American Journal of Epidemiology* 145, no. 4 (1997): 324–34.

Brounstein, Laura. "I Get Up Every Morning and Smile." *Ladies Home Journal*, May 2004, 116–24.

Carr, Bruce R., Richard E. Blackwell. Textbook of Reproductive Medicine. Norwalk, Conn.: Appleton & Lange, 1995.

Cargill, S.L., J.R. Carey, H.G. Muller, G. Anderson. "Age of Ovary Determines Remaining Life Expectancy in Old Ovariectomized Mice." *Aging Cell* 2, no. 3 (2003):185–90.

CDC. "Ten Great Public Health Achievements—United States, 1900-1999." *MMWR Weekly* 48, no. 12 (1999): 241–43. Retrieved from http://www.cdc.gov/epo/mmwr/preview/mmwrhtml/00056796.htm.

CDC National Center for Health Statistics. "Deaths: Preliminary Data for 2002." *NVSR* 52, no. 13: 48.

Confino, E., X. Zhang, R.R. Kazer. "GnRHa Flare and IVF Pregnancy Rates." *International Journal of Gynaecology and Obstetrics* 85, no. 1 (2004): 36–9.

Copperman, A.B. "Antagonists in Poor-Responder Patients." *Fertility and Sterility* 80, suppl 1:S16–24; discussion S32–4 (2003).

Copperman, A.B., T. Mukherjee, B. Sandler, L. Grunfeld, P.A. Bergh, R.T. Scott. "Pre-treatment With Oral Contraceptive Pill Improves Outcome in IVF Cycles of Poor-Responders Using the GNRH Antagonist." *Fertility and Sterility* 80, no. 3 (2003): S108 Abstracts.

Department of Health and Human Services, Food and Drug Administration, Center for Biologics Evaluation and Research, Biological Response Modifiers Advisory Committee. Open Session. Meeting #32 transcript. Thursday, May 9, 2002. Hilton Hotel Gaithersburg, MD.

Domar, A.D. "Impact of Psychological Factors on Dropout Rates in Insured Infertility Patients." *Fertility and Sterility* 81, no. 2 (2004): 271–3.

Domar, A.D., D. Clapp, E.A. Slawsby, J. Dusek, B. Kessel, M. Freizinger. "Impact of Group Psychological Interventions on Pregnancy Rates in infertile women." *Fertility and Sterility* 73, no. 4 (2000): 805–11.

Domar, A.D., P.C. Zuttermeister, R. Friedman. "The Psychological Impact of Infertility: A Comparison With Patients With Other Medical Conditions." *Journal of Psychosomatic Obstetrics and Gynaecology* 14, suppl. (1993): 45–52.

Select Bibliography

Donnez, J., M.M. Dolmans, D. Demylle, P. Jadoul, C. Pirard, J. Squifflet, B. Martinez-Madrid, A. Van Langendonckt. "Livebirth After Orthotopic Transplantation of Cryopreserved Ovarian Tissue." *The Lancet* 364, no. 9441 (September 24, 2004): 5000.

Eroglu, A., M. Toner, T.L. Toth. "Beneficial Effect of Microinjected Trehalose on the Cryosurvival of Human Oocytes." *Fertility and Sterility* 77, no. 1 (2002): 152–8.

Fabbri, R., E. Porcu, T. Marsella, G. Rocchetta, S. Venturoli, C. Flamigni,. "Human Oocyte Cryopreservation: New Perspectives Regarding Oocyte Survival." *Human Reproduction* 16, no. 3 (2001): 411–6.

Fakuda, M., K. Fakuda, Andersen C. Yiding, A.G. Byskov. "Anovulations in an Ovary During Two Menstrual Cycles Enhance the Pregnancy Potential of Oocytes Matured in That Ovary During the Following Tthird Cycle." *Human Reproduction* 14, no. 1 (1999): 96–100.

Falcone, T., M. Attaran, M.A. Bedaiwy, J.M. Goldberg. "Ovarian Function Preservation in the Cancer Patient." *Fertility and Sterility* 81, no. 2 (2004): 243–57.

Ferin, M. "Clinical Review 105: Stress and the Reproductive Cycle." *Journal of Clinical Endocrinology and Metabolism* 84, no. 6 (1999): 1768–74.

Galli, R.L., B. Shukitt-Hale, K.A. Youdim, J.A. Joseph. "Fruit Polyphenolics and Brain Aging: Nutritional Interventions Targeting Age-Related Neuronal and Behavioral Deficits." *Annals of the NY Academy of Science* 959 (2002): 128–32.

Geijsen, N., M. Horoschak, K. Kim, J. Gribnau, K. Eggan, G.Q. Daley. "Derivation of Embryonic Germ Cells and Male Gametes From Embryonic Stem Cells." *Nature* 427 (2004): 148–54. Epub December, 10, 2003.

Hamilton, B.E., J.A. Martin, P.D. Sutton. "Births: Preliminary Data for 2002." Centers for Disease Control and Prevention, National Vital Statistics Reports 51, no. 11 (2003).

Hassan, M.A., S.R. Killick. "Negative Lifestyle Is Associated With a Significant Reduction in Fecundity." *Fertility and Sterility* 81, no. 2 (2004): 384–92.

Hawkes, K. "Grandmothers and the Evolution of Human Longevity." *American Journal of Human Biology* 15, no. 3 (2003): 380–400.

Hawkes, K., J.F. O'Connell, N.G. Blurton Jones, H. Alvarez, E.L. Charnov. "Grandmothering, Menopause, and the Evolution of Human Life Histories." Proceedings of the National Academy of Sciences USA, February 1998.

Hewlett, Sylvia A. *Creating a Life: Professional Women and the Quest for Children*. New York: Talk Miramax Books, 2002.

———. "Executive Women and the Myth of Having it All." *Harvard Business Review* (April 2002): 5–11.

213

Hubner, K., G. Fuhrmann, L.K. Christenson, J. Kehler, R. Reinbold, R. De La Fuente, J. Wood, J.F. Strauss, M. Boiani, H.R. Scholer. "Derivation of Oocytes From Mouse Embryonic Stem Cells." *Science* 300, no. 5623 (2003): 1251–6. Published online May 1, 2003.

Immulite 2000, FSH (PIL2KFS-8, 2003-08-14), p. 4. Instructional booklet.

Jacqz-Aigrain, E., D. Zhang, G. Maillard, D. Luton, J. Andre, J.F. Oury. "Maternal Smoking During Pregnancy and Nicotine and Cotinine Concentrations in Maternal and Neonatal Hair." *International Journal of Obstetrics and Gynaecology* 109, no. 8 (2002): 909–11.

Johnson, Beth."Joan Lunden: A Home Coming." *Good Housekeeping*, September 2003, 161–5.

Jensen, T.K., N.A. Andersen, N.E. Skakkebaek. "Is Human Fertility Declining?" *International Congress Series* 1266 (2004): 32–44.

Johnson, J., J. Canning, T. Kaneko, J.K. Pru, J.L. Tilly. "Germline Stem Cells and Follicular Renewal in the Postnatal Mammalian Ovary." *Nature* 11, no. 428 (2004): 145–50.

Kalb, Claudia, K. Springen, J. Scelfo, E. Pierce. "Should You Have Your Baby Now?" *Newsweek*, August 13, 2003, 40–8.

Keefe, D.L. "Reproductive Aging Is an Evolutionarily Programmed Strategy That No Longer Provides Adaptive Value." *Fertility and Sterility* 70, no. 2 (1998): 204–6.

Keefe, D.L., S. Franco, L. Liu, J. Trimarchi, M. Blasco, S. Weitzen. "Short Telomeres in the Chromosomes of Spare Eggs Predict Poor Prognosis Following in Vitro Fertilization/Embryo Transfer-Toward a Telomere Theory of Reproductive Aging in Women. *Fertility and Sterility* 80, suppl. 3 (2003): 1.

Kong, L.H., Z. Liu, H. Li, L. Zhu, F.Q. Xing. "Pregnancy in a 46-Year-Old Woman After Autologous Granular Cell Mitochondria Transfer." *Di Yi Jun Yi Da Xue Xue Bao* 23, no. 7 (2003): 743–7.

Kono, T., Y. Obata, Q. Wu, K. Niwa, Y. Ono, Y. Yamamoto, E.S. Park, J.S. Seo, H. Ogawa. "Birth of Parthenogenetic Mice That Can Develop to Adulthood." *Nature* 428, no. 6985 (2004): 860–4.

Laufer, N., A. Simon, A. Samueloff, H. Yaffe, A. Milwidsky, Y. Gielchinsky. "Successful Spontaneous Pregnancies in Women Older Than 45 Years." *Fertility and Sterility* 81, no. 5 (2004): 1328–32.

Levi, A.J., M.F. Raynault, P.A. Bergh, M.R. Drews, B.T. Miller, R.T. Scott, Jr. "Reproductive Outcome in Patients With Diminished Ovarian Reserve." *Fertility and Sterility* 76, no. 4 (2001): 666–9.

Liebmann-Smith, Joan, Jacqueline Nardi Egan, John Stangel. *The Unofficial Guide to Overcoming Infertility*. New York: Hungry Minds, 1999.

Liu, J., G. Lu, Y. Qian, Y. Mao, W. Ding. "Pregnancies and Births Achieved From in Vitro Matured Oocytes Retrieved From Poor Responders Undergoing Stimulation in Vitro Fertilization Cycles." *Fertility and Sterility* 80, no. 2 (2003): 447–9.

Liu, L., J.R. Trimarchi, P. Navarro, M.A. Blasco, D.L. Keefe. "Oxidative Stress Contributes to Arsenic-Induced Telomere Attrition, Chromosome Instability and Apoptosis." *Journal of Biological Chemistry* 278, no. 34 (2003): 31998–32004.

Liu, L., J.R. Trimarchi, P.J. Smith, D. Keefe. "Mitochondrial Dysfunction Leads to Telomere Attrition and Genomic Instability." *Aging Cell* 1, no. 1 (2002): 40–46.

Lunden, Joan. Interview with Larry King. *Larry King Live*. CNN, February 12, 2003. Retrieved from http://www.cnn.com/TRANSCRIPTS/0302/12/lkl.00.html.

Lutz, W., B. O'Neill, S. Scherbov, Vienna Institute of Demography, Austrian Academy of Sciences. "Europe's Population at a Turning Point." *Science* 299 (2003): 1991–2.

Muasher, S.J., S. Oehninger, S. Simonetti, J. Matta, L.M. Ellis, H.C. Liu, G.S. Jones, Z. Rosenwaks. "The Value of Basal and/or Stimulated Serum Gonadotropin Levels in Prediction of Stimulation Response and in Vitro Fertilization Outcome." *Fertility and Sterility* 50, no. 2 (1988): 298–307.

National Center for Health Statistics (NCHS). "U.S. Life Expectancy at All-Time High, But Infant Mortality Increases," press release, February 11, 2004.

Navot, D., Z. Rosenwaks, E.J. Margalioth. "Prognostic Assessment of Female Fecundity." *Lancet* 2, no. 8560 (1987): 645–7.

Nightingale, Stuart L., Associate Commissioner for Health Affairs, Food and Drug Administration, Department of Health and Human Services. Letter to institutional review boards confirming the FDA's jurisdiction over clinical research utilizing cloning technology. October 26, 1998.

Oktay, K., E. Buyuk, L. Veeck, N. Zaninovic, K. Xu, T. Takeuchi, M. Opsahl, Z. Rosenwaks. "Embryo Development After Heterotopic Transplantation of Cryopreserved Ovarian Tissue." *Lancet* 363, no. 9412 (2004): 837–40.

Olivius, C., B. Friden, G. Borg, C. Bergh. "Why Do Couples Discontinue in Vitro Fertilization Treatment? A Cohort Study." *Fertility and Sterility* 81, no. 2 (2004): 258–61.

Packer, C., M. Tatar, A. Collins. "Reproductive Cessation in Female Mammals." *Nature* 392, no. 6678 (1998): 807–11.

Packer, Criag. "Why Menopause?" *Natural History* 107, no. 6 (1998): 24–6.

Palermo, G.D., T. Takeuchi, Z. Rosenwaks. "Oocyte-Induced Haploidization." *Reproductive BioMed Online* 4, no. 3 (2002): 237–42.

215

Paulson, R.J., R. Boostanfar, P. Saadat, E. Mor, D.E. Tourgeman, C.C. Slater, M.M. Francis, J.K. Jain. "Pregnancy in the Sixth Decade of Life: Obstetric Outcomes in Women of Advanced Reproductive Age." *Journal of the American Medical Association* 288, no. 18 (2002): 2320–3.

Pavlik, E.J., P.D. DePriest, H.H. Gallion, F.R. Ueland, M.B. Reedy, R.J. Kryscio, J.R. van Nagell, Jr. "Ovarian Volume Related to Age." *Gynecologic Oncology* 77, no. 3 (2000): 410–2.

Perls, T.T., L. Alpert, R.C. Fretts. "Middle-Aged Mothers Live Longer." *Nature* 389, no. 6647 (1997): 133.

Perls, T.T., R.C. Fretts. "The Evolution of Menopause and Human Life Span." *Annals of Human Biology* 28, no. 3 (2001): 237–45.

Practice Committee of the American Society for Reproductive Medicine. "Aging and Infertility in Women." *Fertility and Sterility* 82, suppl 1 (2004): 102–106.

Resolve, The National Infertility Association, with Diane Aronson, executive director. *Resovling Infertility*. New York: HarperCollins Publishers Inc., 1999.

Rosenwaks, Z. "We Still Can't Stop the Biological Clock." Op-Ed, *New York Times*, June 24, 2000.

Saretzki, G., T. von Zglinicki. "Replicative Senescence as a Model of Aging: The Role of Oxidative Stress and Telomere Shortening—An Overview." [Article in German] *Z Gerontol Geriatr* 32, no. 2 (1999): 69–75.

Scheffer, G.J., F. Broekmans, M. Dorland, J. Habbema, W.N. Looman, E.R. te Velde. "Antral Follicle Counts by Transvaginal Ultrasonography Are Related to Age in Women With Proven Natural Fertility." *Fertility and Sterility* 72, no. 5 (1999): 845–51.

Schwartz-Bickenbach, D., B. Schulte-Hobein, S. Abt, C. Plum, H. Nau. "Smoking and Passive Smoking During Pregnancy and Early Infancy: Effects on Birth Weight, Lactation Period, and Cotinine Concentrations in Mother's Milk and Infant's Urine." *Toxicology Letters* 35, no. 1 (1987): 73–81.

Serono Reproductive Health, A History of Fertility Advances, 2003 Serono, Inc., CD.

Smolowe, Jill, and N. Stoynoff. "Teaming With Love." *People*, March 10, 2003, 88–94.

Soules, M.R., American Society for Reproductive Medicine. "The story behind the American Society for Reproductive Medicine's prevention of infertility campaign." *Fertility and Sterility* 80, no. 2 (2003): 295–9.

Stillman, Robert J. "Smoking and Infertility," Prevention of Infertility Source Document, submitted to the ASRM Prevention of Infertility Committee, http://www.protectyourfertility.com/docs/smoking_infertility.doc.

Tarin, J., J. Ten, F.J. Vendrell, M.N. de Oliveira, A. Cano. "Effects of maternal ageing and dietary antioxidant supplementation on ovulation, fertilization and embryo development in vitro in the mouse." *Reproduction Nutrition Development* 38, no. 5 (1998): 499–508.

Tarlatzis, B.C., L. Zepiridis, G. Grimbizis, J. Bontis. "Clinical Management of Low Ovarian Response to Stimulation for IVF: A Systematic Review." *Human Reproduction Update* 9, no. 1 (2003): 61–76.

Tarlatzis, B.C., L. Zepiridis. "Perimenopausal Conception." *Annals of the NY Academy of Science* 997 (2003): 93–104.

Tiegs, Cheryl. Interview with Larry King. *Larry King Live*, CNN, July 14, 2000. Retrieved from http://www-cgi.cnn.com/TRANSCRIPTS/0007/14/lkl.00.html>.

Toner, J.P. "Age = Egg Quality, FSH Level = Egg Quantity." *Fertility and Sterility* 79, no. 3 (2003): 491.

———. "Ovarian Reserve, Female Age and the Chance for Successful Pregnancy." *Minerva Ginecol* 55, no. 5(2003): 399–406.

U.S. Bureau of the Census. *Centenarians in the United States*. P23-199, Washington D.C.

U.S. Congress. House. *Medicare Infertility Coverage Act of 2003*. 108th Cong., 1st sess., 2003. H.R. 969.

———. House. *Equity in Fertility Coverage Act of 2003*. 108th Cong., 1st sess., 2003. H.R. 1852.

———. House. *Family Building Act of 2003*. 108th Cong., 1st sess., 2003. H.R. 3024.

Van Rooij, I.A., L.F. Bansci, F.J. Broekmans, C.W. Looman, J.D. Habbema, E.R. te Velde. "Women Older Than 40 Years of Age and Those With Elevated Follicle Stimulating Hormone Levels Differ in Poor Response Rate and Embryo Quality in Vitro Fertilization." *Fertility and Sterility* 79, no. 3 (2003): 482–8.

Willcox, B.J., D.C. Willcox, M. Suzuki. "Evidence-based Extreme Longevity: The Case of Okinawa, Japan." Okinawa Centenarian Study. 2001 Scientific abstract of research presented at the Presidential Poster Session of the American Geriatrics Society Annual Meeting, www.okinawaprogram.com/evidence.html.

INDEX

ABOUT THE AUTHOR

Cara Birrittieri is an award-winning television reporter who covered health and medicine in Boston and has reported extensively on reproduction issues. Her awards include an Emmy nomination, the Health & Science Journalist's Award from the American Heart Association, the Sword of Hope Award from the Amercian Cancer Society, the Award of Excellence from the American Medical Writer's Association, and an AAAS Science Journalism Award. Since undergoing her own battle with her biological clock, she has appeared on many health news segments involving fertility. She resides outside Boston, Massachusetts, with her husband, 5-year-old son, and infant daughter.